The Journey Home from Trauma

A Study of Complementary Treatment

Dr. Terry J. Martin PsyD, LCSW, DCSW

www.journeysthroughlife.com

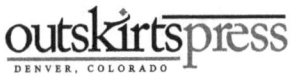

outskirtspress

DENVER, COLORADO

Dedication

Many people deserve my heartfelt appreciation for their support and contribution to the successful completion of this study. I thank my parents, and my beautiful Ilio, Mitzi who offer me their spiritual support from Heaven every day of my life. Mahalo Nui Loa goes out to my family, and my Ohana in Hawaii. I express my gratitude to my dear friend Corline (Corkie), and especially Gene who are always there to listen, support and help me process my frustrations and stay in the Now. They have all been immensely helpful and supportive to me on this journey.

A special Mahalo Nui Loa goes out to Mr. Christopher M. Slavens MSW, MAJ (ret) Hawaii Army National Guard and Iraq Combat War Veteran who has been supportive, and always willing to offer his personal insight as a combat Veteran. His contributions significantly added to this study, and he truly exemplifies what a true hero/Veteran is, and I am honored to know him, and to work with him serving our service members and Veterans.

Lastly, this study is dedicated to all of the military service members, (active duty, guard, reservist), and Veterans that I have been honored and blessed to help treat over the years in my clinical practice, and who have sacrificed so much to protect our freedom as a nation. May all of them always get the support, help, and respect they have earned and deserve from our country, the United States of America.

Praise for
The Journey Home from Trauma
A Study of Complementary Treatment

Dr. Terry J. Martin, a psycho/therapist who has provided direct clinical practice to active duty service members and combat Veterans throughout his exemplary career, and has been practicing and researching meditation for many years. The thoroughness of Dr. Martin's research makes this book a must have for those considering or currently using meditation in their clinical practice with those who have experienced traumas, especially military related traumas. This book covers all the relevant topics related to transcendental meditation, i.e., personal health, contentedness, relationships, spirituality, peace, centeredness and self-actualization, in a clear, concise, stimulating and informative manner. Please consider this book a reader-friendly introduction for anyone considering using meditation in their clinical practice with service members and Veterans.

JASON L. DURR, LCSW, BCD
CPT, MS
UNITED STATES ARMY RESERVES

Dr. Martin has done an amazing job reviewing all the literature on meditation and its effectiveness on military members facing trauma. As a practicing transcendental meditator and counselor, I can attest to the benefits this book thoroughly covers. Dr. Martin has done the research work for you and compiled all the studies into one book. Not only will this book save you time and money, it will help you help your clients reach their healing goals without medication. This book is a must have for every counselor's tool box!

Dr. Elaine A. Kono Ed.D
Chief Master Sergeant
United States Air Force (Retired)

Foreword

The importance of this work cannot be overstated. Not only for the lives of the Veterans themselves, but also for the lives of all of those who are related to, love and care for the combat Veterans of this nation. Inability to transition home from war is something that every generation of combat Veterans has experienced. If history has taught us anything, it's that Combat Stress Injuries do not heal without time and energy being put directly on healing from them. One does not simply "get over it."

Having returned in January of 2006 from an 18 month military deployment including a year-long tour of duty in Iraq, I had no idea how profoundly my life, and the lives of my family, would be impacted as a result of the changes we all went through over those many months. The next years after redeploying were incredibly difficult for me, my kids and my spouse as I struggled with anger, stress, anxiety, sleeplessness, and isolation. I knew I felt different and believed that if I just stayed busy enough and gave myself time, I would get better in time. I really had no real idea how much I was hurting myself or the ones I loved with this pattern of thought. The reality was that time alone only made things worse.

Much has been written lately about the difficult effects that military deployments have on those who serve and on their families who serve right along with them. For the last four and a half years that I have worked with transitioning military service members, Veterans and their families, as well as working on my own transition and recovery, one of the most surprising things I have found is not just how little society knows about these war Veterans but, amazingly, how little we Veterans know about ourselves while in transition.

Combat stress injuries take many forms. As a result of over 14 years of war that our country has been actively engaged in since 9-11, the less than 1% of Americans who make up the global war on terrorism Veteran pool have borne the brunt of these effects of prolonged stress, trauma and transition. Extraordinarily high divorce rates, unprecedentedly high suicide rates and chronic homelessness all point to the difficulty that this newest generation of combat Veterans is having in making the transition home.

My journey with Transcendental Meditation (TM) started just over a year ago and the effects have been immediately positive and lasting. Increased ability to relax, regulate my thoughts and emotions, and increased ability to get to and remain asleep are among the greatest increases in my quality of life after discovering the gift of TM.

One of the most interesting things that I have noticed since starting on this TM journey is the stigma associated with the knowledge and practice of TM. Not unlike the stigma associated with seeking help with mental health while in the military, it appears to me that many of the people I have encouraged to try TM look at it as too strange, different or weird to even give it a try. People often mistakenly associate TM with a religious belief or mystic practice and are therefore unwilling to even consider it. When I explain that TM is simply exercise for your mind that allows it to relax and be free, many times people have a difficult time accepting this perspective.

Considering that the knowledge of TM is thousands of years old, It is my hope that people who read this body of work approach it with an open mind and really consider the power that such a widely studied and highly successful practice that TM is on helping people to improve their mental and physical health and thus improve the quality of their daily lives.

Lastly, it is important for me to acknowledge the author of this important study, Dr. Terry J. Martin. I will forever be grateful to him as my friend, colleague and mentor for introducing me to the practice of Transcendental Meditation, and for believing in me enough to trust me with the responsibility of assisting our returning combat Veterans. He gave me a chance when I was not necessarily the obvious choice, and for that I will always do my best to honor his trust and continue to work to pay his gift to me forward. His faith in me has been instrumental in finally embracing my own transition home, and in helping to guide others back to a more peaceful, joyful and fulfilled post war existence.

Christopher M. Slavens, MSW

MAJ (ret) HIARNG

Iraq War Veteran

Prologue

Scope of Study

This study examines the question of meditation as a complementary treatment for PTSD and anxiety symptoms, and recommends the most effective form of meditation technique to reduce symptoms.

Results demonstrate that meditation is highly effective in treating a varied population suffering from PTSD and anxiety, and that meditation can have a positive effect. Included is also a review and evaluation of current empirical research concerning open, focused, and transcendent meditation techniques, to determine if they are helpful in treating PTSD, and anxiety symptoms.

The study identifies the effects of these various meditation techniques, and the benefits they offer to an individual suffering from PTSD and anxiety. It also addresses the effects on positive and negative affect, attention, happiness, and health-related behaviors that are affected by stress, pain, and trauma.

The evidence from this study is useful for clinicians and patients in making decisions about the best available options for stress reduction. Meditation can be defined as a family of practices that train attention and awareness, usually with the objective of fostering psychological and spiritual wellbeing and maturity. Meditation does this by training and bringing mental processes under greater voluntary control, and directing them in beneficial ways.

This control is used to cultivate specific mental qualities such as concentration and calm, and emotions such as joy, love, and compassion. Through greater awareness, a clearer understanding of oneself and one's relationship to the world develops (Hofman, Grossman, & Hinton, 2011).

Contents

LIST OF TABLES

LIST OF FIGURES

Chapter 1

Introduction to the Problem

The President of the United States, Barack Obama, ordered the Department of Defense to reduce the U.S. combat forces in Iraq and Afghanistan beginning in 2011 (Facts and Figures on Drawdown in Iraq, 2010). The order directed the Department of Defense to remove all military ground combat forces exiting Iraq by 2011/2012 and Afghanistan in 2014 (Facts, 2010). The President's plan outlined that a small number of U.S. forces might be left behind once all of the combat forces left. However, the Iraqi government did not want any U.S. troops left in their country (Facts, 2010).

As of 2011, 1,318,510 Operation Enduring Freedom (OEF), Operation Iraqi Freedom (OIF) and Operation New Dawn (OND) veterans (see Table 1) had left active duty and became eligible for health care since 2002 (Office of Public Health, 2011). The demographic characteristics of the OEF/OIF/OND veteran population utilizing Veterans Administration (VA) health care are 87.4% male and 11.9% female (Fonata, Rosenheck, & Desi, 2010).

A total of 349,786 patients have received a diagnosis of a possible mental disorder since 2002 (Office, 2011). The numbers of OEF/OIF veterans who have been diagnosed with PTSD and have been seen at a VA Healthcare Center since 2002 is 202,056 according to the U.S. Department of Public Health (2011) and Shea, Vujanovic, Mansfield, Sevin, and Liu (2010). As the OEF/OIF veterans return home from battle, many of them face the individual and interpersonal aftereffects of duty-related trauma (Klosterman, Rielage, Hoyt, & Renshaw, 2010). The OEF and OIF wars have brought heightened awareness of combat-related PTSD. Among veterans, mental disorders such as combat-related PTSD are epidemic (Seal, Bertentahl, Miner, Sauank, & Marmar, 2007; U.S. Department of Public Health, 2011).

Table 1

Post-911 War Veterans by Birth Year

Veteran Birth Years	Totals	Percentage
1980-1995	597,285	45.30%
1970-1979	346,768	26.30%
1960-1969	276,887	21.00%
1950-1959	84,384	6.40%
1926-1949	13,185	1.00%

Note. Table 1 represents the breakdown, by birth year, of the veterans of the post-911 global war on terrorism (Office of Public Health, 2011).

The Department of Veterans Affairs estimates that 30% of U.S. soldiers deployed to Afghanistan and Iraq since 2001 are said to suffer from PTSD. PTSD symptoms are among the precipitating factors that have made suicide the leading cause of death among active duty soldiers (Shiner, 2011; U.S. Department of Public Health, 2011).

There are significant mental health issues reported by service members who were deployed to Iraq or Afghanistan. The President of the United States ended the war in Iraq (OIF), and then subsequently removed all military operations. The U.S. is now only engaged in the conflict in Afghanistan (OEF). The current conflict as of 2012 is referred to by the Department of Defense as OEF and OND. OND is focused on peacekeeping activities within Iraq post-withdrawal.

In 2012, many war veterans returned from multiple deployments. They returned to their life routines with their families and picked up where they left off in their daily life struggles. Everything in their lives was put on hold for 12-18 months while they were on deployments until they returned home.

They would talk to their families on video (Skype) often. They would hear about all of the problems their families were struggling with, and they felt powerless to help them resolve their problems because of their own physical absence from their families; this only added to their high stress levels (Grosswald & Yellin, 2011).

When they returned from their deployment, many of them had difficulty with their transition and assimilation with their families and their communities in society. They were not the same as the family had remembered before they deployed when life was more predictable (Collinge, Kahn, & Soltysik, 2012).

Surviving a traumatic event such as combat, an earthquake, or a violent personal assault can be psychologically devastating. On one hand, individuals would feel alive, but their experiences haunted them through flashbacks or nightmares. They were continually on edge, easily startled, and might feel intense guilt, or emotional numbness. Their diagnosis was PTSD (Wood, Wiederhold, & Spira, 2010).

Meditation can help someone diagnosed with anxiety because it can help to eliminate the source of stress in the mind and the body, and provide profound relaxation that helps the body to naturally dissolve deeply rooted stresses (Horowitz, 2010). It is a family of practices that train attention and awareness, usually with the objective of fostering psychological and spiritual wellbeing and maturity. Meditation does this by training and bringing one's mental processes under greater voluntary control, and directing them in beneficial ways (Horowitz, 2010).

This control is used to cultivate specific mental qualities such as concentration and calm, and emotions such as joy, love, and compassion. Through greater awareness, a clearer understanding of oneself and one's relationship to the world develops. Thus, a deeper and more accurate knowledge of consciousness and reality manifests (Marchand, 2012).

To treat stress and stress-related conditions, as well as to promote health, meditation is used widely by both clinical populations and the public. There are hospitals and programs now that are offering courses in meditation for patients who are seeking alternative or additional methods to relieve ailments or to promote health (Meditation, 2013).

I suggest that with the ever-increasing usage of meditation across a large spectrum of health conditions; examining the effects of meditation, the types of meditation techniques, conditions for which they are efficacious, and any mechanisms of action are important for patients, clinicians, and policymakers to know. Meditation offers a rich and complex field of study. Over the past 40 years, over 600 research studies have demonstrated numerous significant findings including changes in psychological, physiological, and transpersonal realms (Horowitz, 2010).

Background of the Problem

Even though it is common to experience PTSD symptoms following trauma, most individuals will not develop the full syndrome. Early or mild symptoms often resolve without the need for treatment (McLay, Loeffler, & Wynn, 2013, p. 39). Many of the military personnel who have been deployed worked as interpreters and were instructed by their leaders to focus on building relationships with the local population as part of their mission (Grosswald & Yellin, 2011). The non-military locals often viewed the American military as a foreign invader in Iraq and Afghanistan. They sometimes used their own children and other family members as armed weapons to fight the invaders (Roberts, Engel, Cordova, & Jonas, 2011). They would strap improvised explosive devices to their bodies, and would walk into a crowd fully aware of what they were doing. The U.S. military personnel were unaware of their lethal intent and were injured or killed when the suicide bombers would detonate their bombs (Grosswald & Yellin, 2011).

To the soldier, survival meant to trust no one. Paranoia, hypervigilance, anxiety, and sleep disorders became the norm of the soldiers' behavior in their daily lives. The adoption and adaptation of these survival behaviors has helped them to survive their war-torn physical environment, but it comes at an enormous emotional cost because it has led to a whole array of emotional angst for these soldiers when they return home (Roberts et al., 2011).

The numerous deployments have only exacerbated their angst and have helped to increase the possibility of experiencing a combat-related physical injury(s) and/or a traumatic event(s). These psychological issues and physical injuries have had a negative effect on their families and on their lives. The signature wounds of these wars have been traumatic brain injury and PTSD (Tanielani & Jaycox, 2008).

Statement of the Problem

The problem is that it is not known if the practice of meditation is efficacious as a complementary treatment/co-therapy to treat PTSD symptoms in veterans, and what, if any, is the most effective form of meditation technique that can help to reduce and/or eliminate PTSD symptoms.

Purpose of the Study

Numerous studies have been conducted that suggest that those veterans diagnosed with PTSD have seen a lowering of symptoms and an improvement in their focus through the practice of meditation. It seems to produce its effects through a variety of mechanisms, and it has been shown to improve dramatically one's ability to retain new information (Borman et al. 2005).

The purpose of this theoretical study is to evaluate and review the research to determine whether meditation is efficacious as a complementary treatment for veterans diagnosed with PTSD/anxiety. Is meditation an effective complementary treatment for PTSD with other populations, and what meditation technique(s) shows the greatest potential to treat PTSD anxiety symptoms (Cukor, Spitalnick, Difede, Rizzo, & Rothbaum, 2009)?

Theoretical Framework

Many Americans use complementary and alternative medicine (CAM) in pursuit of health and wellbeing. The 2007 National Health Interview Survey shows that approximately 38% of adults use CAM (Meditation, 2013). The need for doing more research on CAM is important now. Over the past nine years, over 2 million American soldiers have served in Iraq and Afghanistan, and over 15% of them have met the diagnostic criteria for PTSD (Borman, Golshan, Thorp, Wetherell, & Lang, 2009).

The basis for this project is to investigate the efficacy of meditation technique(s), and determine if they need to be considered as a complementary treatment intervention in conjunction with conventional treatments, and not to view meditation as an alternative treatment in place of conventional medicine, but to be aware that mediation can be considered a prescribed complementary treatment intervention along with other conventional treatments for PTSD/anxiety symptoms.

There is frequently an increase in mental health concerns as an effect of military-related traumatic events, and these problems often increase in the ensuing months following a deployment from battle (Collinge et al., 2012). My goal was to present a well-balanced discussion regarding the clinical efficacy of military veterans by comparing and contrasting with others who have used meditation as a complementary treatment intervention to help them manage their various major psychological symptoms of anxiety (Brooks, & Scarano, 1985)

The current meditation-based interventions are considered complementary therapies, not conventional medicine. The three operational definitions of meditation are: (a) object-*focused* or concentrative meditation, (b) *open*-monitoring or moment-to-moment meditation, and (c) *transcendent* meditation (Borman et al., 2009, p. 2).

There is a discussion of the theoretical and empirical evidence that meditation works by inducing changes in psychological capacities such as emotion regulation and self-regulation, and through repeated induction of specific mental states such as love or meta-cognitive awareness.

Research Questions

The research questions advanced in this study are:

- RQ 1: Does meditation help in treating PTSD/anxiety symptoms?

- RQ 2: Does it help in decreasing PTSD/anxiety symptoms?

- RQ 3: Does meditation contribute to an increase in positive physiological health?

- RQ 4: Of the three meditation techniques reviewed (i.e., open, focused, and transcendent), which technique will be shown to be the most effective in reducing PTSD/anxiety symptoms in veterans or other populations?

Importance of the Study

The significance of the results from the research is critical to helping to design and develop an inclusive and comprehensive standard complementary treatment intervention model, one that can be used widely by veterans and others, and adopted by healthcare practitioners as being a viable intervention to employ within an array of private and public healthcare settings to help in the treatment of PTSD symptoms, as well as facilitating good health.

The use of meditation in the treatment of PTSD will have a positive effect on wellbeing, and have a positive effect on reducing symptoms of PTSD such as insomnia, depression, anxiety, emotional numbness, migraine headaches, high blood pressure, pain, and many other related symptoms (Horowitz, 2010; Jakupcak, Wagner, Paulson, Varra, & McFall, 2010).

The number of individuals using meditation is steadily increasing as they are seeking complementary treatment choices to address and possibly alleviate a number of their physical and emotional issues. There is a desire expressed by many veterans and others who would like to integrate a more holistic and philosophical approach to their health care (Meditation, 2013).

Veterans report that adopting a holistic approach helps to provide them greater control and offer them more options to consider in their individual healthcare treatment process(s) (Strauss & Lang, 2012). Meditation could be helpful to veterans and others who are suffering from anxiety and to help offer another tool for health care providers to use (Simpson et al., 2007; Waelde et al. 2008). This supposition could help health care policymakers to design better health care policies that will be comprehensive and inclusive of a number of complementary treatment alternatives available to health care consumers. This process can have an important impact on what is available to both the public and private healthcare settings in the United States.

The different techniques of meditative intervention discussed in this study can be considered as ways to reduce symptomatology and improve the quality of life for individuals with PTSD. Like all anxiety disorders, PTSD is characterized by inappropriate triggering of the fight-flight response, the body's automatic response to danger (Lang et al., 2012, p. 768). The practice of meditation holds great therapeutic promise and application as a set of techniques for dissolving stress, and self-actualization including autonomy, creativity, inner satisfaction, focus, alertness, and productivity (Borman et al., 2009).

In a state of meditation, only mental techniques appear to generate a unique and reproducible state of physiology in which the mind displays increased alertness without an object of perception while the body gains an unusually deep state of rest (Coppola & Spector, 2009; Jevning, Wallace, & Beidebach, 1992).

Scope of the Study

The rationale of this study is to discover how meditation practice (technique) compares to other methods of treating PTSD symptoms. To what degree, if any, does mediation practice (technique) complement treatment intervention in reducing PTSD symptoms in veterans or others?

There were a comprehensive review and evaluation conducted on empirical research concerning open, focused, and transcendent meditations to determine if they are helpful in treating and/or eliminating PTSD anxiety symptoms with this population and others.

As mentioned earlier, meditation is simply a collection of practices that help with training one's attention and awareness. The objective is to facilitate psychological and spiritual wellbeing and maturity. It accomplishes this by helping one to bring one's mental processes under greater voluntary control and helping to focus them in valuable ways (Horowitz, 2010).

When an individual is able to gain control, it can be used by him or her to develop particular mental qualities such as concentration and calm, and emotions such as joy, love, and compassion. Through the development of awareness, there emerges a lucid insight into oneself, and their relationship to the world develops. Thus, a deeper and more accurate knowledge of consciousness and reality manifests (Marchand, 2012).

Meditation is widely accepted as a mind-body technique that helps one maintain holistic health and wellness. Research studies present strong outcomes indicating that meditation is a "safe and effective complementary therapy for treating a variety of conditions, and is very effective in treating the psychological effects of chronic illness (anxiety), and the pain effects that are not often addressed in conventional treatments" (Horowitz, 2010, p. 227). I will summarize these findings regarding the recent research on the efficacy of meditation as a complementary treatment for PTSD symptoms, and will draw comparisons and contrasts.

Definitions of Terms

Complementary medicine—a group of diagnostic and therapeutic disciplines that are used together with conventional medicine (Libby, Pilver, & Desai, 2011).

Meditation—a practice of concentrated focus upon a sound, object, visualization, the breath, movement, or attention itself in order to increase awareness of the present moment, reduce stress, promote relaxation, and enhance personal and spiritual growth. It can benefit people with, or without, acute medical illness or stress, and people who meditate regularly have been shown to feel less anxiety and depression (Lang et al., 2012).

PTSD is categorized among the anxiety disorders in the *Diagnostic and Statistical Manual of Mental Disorders* fourth edition text revision. It occurs in the aftermath of a traumatic event. Examples are combat, rape, and natural disasters, and are usually diagnosed after six months after the traumatic event.

There are three major types of PTSD symptoms; the traumatized person generally (a) develops a heightened startle response, (b) is vulnerable to having memories of the trauma come flooding back into his or her mind at unexpected moments (flashbacks), or (c) will go to great lengths to avoid thinking about the trauma (First, Frances, & Pincus, 2002).

A *veteran* is a person who served in the active military, navy, or air service, and who was discharged or released under conditions other than dishonorable (Code of Federal Regulation, 2013), and also who is receiving inpatient and outpatient healtcare at a VA Medical Center as a veteran.

Summary and Organization

Research studies, methods, and procedures were summarized; the methodology used and related literature were reviewed and considered as well as factors that contribute to and identify any limitations in the research. The review examined research studies that have used either an active control, attention control, or education control that can reliably control for placebo effects such as the expectation of benefit and attention. This focus will help to provide the superlative indication of whether an intervention shows efficacy due to the intervention as opposed to efficacy due to a nonspecific placebo type effect, and will abet in reducing the outcomes of selection bias and misperception.

The research findings are offered and evaluated in a consistent manner. The summary provides a review for the reader of previous chapters concerning aforementioned information.

It also includes a synopsis of the research findings followed by a Discussion section. There is a review of the reference lists of each included article, relevant review articles, related systematic reviews, as well as a bibliography and appendices included.

Therefore, it may be deduced from the findings that there is a necessity that conducting future research is imperative. It is crucial to highlight the necessity to continue to expand the paradigm from which meditation research is conducted, from a complex, biomedical model to one that includes subjective and transpersonal domains and an essential perception.

Chapter 2: Review of the Literature

The Post-911 Veteran

Vujanovic, Niles, Pietrefesa, Schnertz, and Potter (2011) discussed the increasing rate of returning military personnel presenting to the Veterans Health Administration (VHA) for mental health services related to trauma exposure or PTSD.

Hoget et al. (2004, as cited in Vujanovic et al., 2011) stated that approximately 25.5% of returning veterans who presented to the VHA had met diagnostic criteria for PTSD, and they also had significant impairments in interpersonal relationships and occupational functioning (Wolf, & Abell, 2003).

Schnurr et al. (2010) stated that these wars and their related events have had a global impact at multiple levels, ranging from individuals to society. There has been an increase in public awareness and recognition of PTSD and other readjustment problems that often result from warzone exposure. This increase in awareness has led to the growth of positive societal responses to these issues (Schnurr et al., 2010, p. 3). As communicated to the American people in a press conference at the White House by President Barack Obama on October 21, 2011, the U.S. military operations were to cease at the end of 2014 in Iraq and Afghanistan. However, they have not. He also stated that the military is scheduled to end its operations in Afghanistan and depart in 2014. However, the U.S. government has signed agreements with the Afghanistan government to keep U.S. soldiers present there through 2019 (Adler, McGurk, Bliese, & Hoge, 2009).

Chard, Schumm, Owens, and Cottingham (2010) stated that the wars in Iraq and Afghanistan have produced a large number of veterans who survived in a war-torn environment that often meant to trust no one, and paranoia, hypervigilance, anxiety, chronic pain, and sleep disorders became the norm of behavior in their daily lives. Because of this stressful environment and the creation of high levels of stress, it actually helped to contribute to their avoidance of injury and death while they were deployed but, unfortunately, it has come at a significant cost to their health.

Schnurr et al. (2010), and Chard et al. (2010) discussed how multiple and prolonged deployments could have been contributing factors that led to these heightened levels of anxiety within the military. This has also helped to add to the numerous combat-related physical injuries and/or traumatic events that the military service members have experienced over the past 10 years or more.

Koenen et al. (2008, as cited in Chard et al., 2010) discussed the significant toll that the numerous deployments and the length of time, which initially began at six months and was extended to eighteen months toward the end of the war in Iraq, has exacted on the service members' wellbeing emotionally and physically.

Chard et al. (2010) discussed the variety of psychological issues and physical injuries, and how they have had an extremely negative effect on their families and on their own lives. The signature wounds of these wars continue to be traumatic brain injury and PTSD (Chard et al., 2010).

The comprehensive literature review will focus on studies that have evaluated and assessed the conventional and complementary treatments for patients diagnosed with PTSD symptoms using both conventional and complementary treatments. These studies involve veterans diagnosed with PTSD and others, who have been prescribed meditation as a complementary treatment intervention.

Existing Treatments for PTSD

Various data that Lang et al. (2012) cite affirm that between one half and one-third of patients who receive empirically supported treatments for PTSD do not fully respond to treatment, and that there is over a 20% dropout rate for any exposure-based prolonged exposure therapy (PE) or cognitive interventions such as cognitive processing therapy (CPT) (Macrodimitris, Hamilton, Backs-Dermott, & Mothersill, 2010).

These high dropout rates are alarming, and warrant a comprehensive review of the research on the significance of meditation practice(s) and their specific techniques in treating PTSD. The findings can be important to help healthcare practitioners determine if the practice of meditation is an empirical, evidence-based, and viable complementary therapeutic treatment option for veterans and others diagnosed with PTSD that they are treating.

Lang et al. (2012) found that CPT and PE therapy are evidence-based treatment therapies that occasionally trigger an acute increase in PTSD symptoms, and contribute to high dropout rates and non-response from patients.

Hamblen, Schnurr, Rosenberg, and Eftekhari (2010) defined PE therapy as involving four primary components:

1. education about reactions to trauma and PTSD,

2. breathing retraining for relaxation,

3. exposure to real world, trauma-related situations that are objectively safe but avoided due to trauma-related distress (in vivo exposure), and

4. exposure to the trauma memory through repeated recounting of the traumatic event (imaginal exposure).

PE has been shown to be effective in working with individuals who have varying traumas. Along with PE, this treatment modality has been recommended by the VHA and the Department of Defense, and incorporated into their practice guidelines for the management of traumatic stress and other corollary symptoms following a traumatic event (U.S. Department of Public Health, 2011).

However, it is not always the best fit for all patients suffering from PTSD. For that reason, it was imperative that this comprehensive review of research be undertaken and that a thorough evaluation of complementary treatment options such as meditation was reviewed. It is hoped that this will begin the process to identify other alternatives that can help address the patients who are currently resistant to western conventional medical treatment.

Hamblen et al., (2010) defined CPT as a 12-session trauma-focused, manualized therapy that is effective for treating PTSD symptoms following traumatic events. In contrast to PE, CPT is recommended to patients who have experienced a whole range of traumatic events including trauma exposure. CPT was originally developed for use with rape and crime victims. Beck and Emery's, (1979) , as cited in Hamblen et al., 2010) cognitive therapy techniques served as a template for CPT. The cognitive process begins with the trauma memory, and it assists the patient to begin to change maladaptive beliefs, feelings, and thoughts that originate from their traumatic event(s).

However, there are concerns as cited in Lang et al. (2012) regarding the use of CPT and PE therapy for the treatment of PTSD. On occasion, these treatment intervention(s) can activate an acute increase in PTSD symptoms, and can help to contribute to high dropout rates among patients. They also lead to a non-response from patients who report they cannot tolerate the treatment(s) of PE or CPT (Monson, Fredman, & Adair, 2008).

Hamblen et al. (2010) made conjecture that cognitive therapies such as PE and CPT are considered first-line treatments for PTSD because they have strong evidence bases. However, even with the strong evidence base of PE, there is concern about the tolerability and the safety of PE for some. Too much anxiety evoked during treatment can sometimes result in sensitization of the patient, and PE treatment might not be considered viable because of this concern. Other psychodynamic methods may be selected instead of PE as alternatives to treat PTSD instead of cognitive processing because of the potential side effect that PE treatment may exacerbate a patient's symptoms of PTSD (Hamblen et al., 2010).

The investigators in these studies endeavored to identify and address the reasons for high treatment dropout rates, and the overall dissatisfaction of patients treated in an inpatient and outpatient setting with conventional western medicine. Their premise reaffirms that complementary therapies such as meditation can offer a viable treatment option for persons with PTSD as being a complementary treatment with conventional treatment. They propose that meditation needs to be made available, and considered as a possible treatment option to offer to patients who do not respond favorably to evidence-based treatments, such as CPT and PE.

In contrast to CPT and PE treatment, Libby et al. (2011) established that a mind-body treatment such as meditation is effective for the regulation of physiological and psychological arousal symptoms of PTSD. Lang et al. (2012) also examined how CPT and, especially PE treatment techniques, sometimes exacerbate the arousal symptoms in patients with PTSD. One of the reasons cited in the study is that PE therapy has the patient focus on reviewing trauma to recover, and this process frequently triggers trauma memories that can become disabling for the patient.

Libby et al. (2011) did not address each of the three techniques of meditation and their efficacy to treat PTSD, but did identify and theorized that the overall practice of meditation as another complementary therapy for patients with PTSD were very effective for symptom abatement, along with others such as relaxation and exercise therapy.

Complementary Alternative Medicine (CAM)

Mental health problems are among the most frequently cited reasons for seeking help from a complementary provider who can offer meditation as a treatment intervention (McLay,

Loeffler, Wynn, & Gary, 2013). McLay, Loeffler, Wynn, and Gary (2013) separated CAM modalities into three categories:

- modalities that fit within the modern conceptualization of medical science,

- modalities that do not fit into this conceptualization, but do not directly challenge it, and

- modalities that challenge established scientific principles.

Interventions such as herbal medications and exercise belong to the first category. Acupuncture, chiropractic, and the three meditation techniques (i.e., open, focused, and transcendent) this study is reviewing fit into the second category of CAM treatment. The third category would consist of certain practices of homeopathy and the idea that a prayer has an effect in those unaware they are being prayed for (Barnes, Bloom, & Nahin 2008).

These definitions of what CAM is, specifically one and two, assist clinicians by offering an array of choices of complementary treatment options that have an empirical basis. They can also be used as complementary meditation in helping to treat a complex disorder such as PTSD.

The combination of conventional and complementary treatment interventions can begin to address the problem of reducing some of the high dropout rates, and dissatisfaction in patients with PTSD that have difficulty tolerating the conventional western medicine interventions being prescribed such as medications, CPT, or PE (Brauser, 2011).

Kroesen, Baldwin, Brooks, and Bell (2002) assessed the growing use of CAM among US military veterans. They wanted to discover why someone would turn to CAM and if the decision was because of his or her dissatisfaction with the conventional care system that he or she had accessed for care. The participants in the study mentioned dissatisfaction with reliance on prescription medications and the lack of holism that exists in conventional medicine. These two dynamics were the precipitating factors that helped to motivate them to seek treatments outside of conventional medicine, such as CAM. Modalities that do not fit into this conceptualization and do not directly challenge medical science such as open, focused, and transcendent meditation, are sought out as possible complementary treatment interventions by patients who are dealing with chronic PTSD symptoms.

They are exhausted, upset, and have become aware of how incomplete conventional healthcare is in providing care to treat their chronic illness. A list of chronic conditions such as headaches, depression, anxiety, insomnia, fatigue, a low threshold for pain, and high blood pressure are often reported by these patients (Kearney, McDermott, Malte, Martinez, & Simpson, 2012). They no longer have any belief in the effectiveness of conventional health care medicine in helping to treat their symptoms (National Institute of Health, 2013).

Recent studies reviewed by Eisenberg et al. (1998, as cited in Kroesen et al., 2002) indicate that there has been an exponential increase of patients seeking out CAM. There has been an increase from 33.8% in 1990 to 42.1% in 1997, and the number of visits that Americans made to CAM providers has increased to 47.3%. These rising statistics are alarming, but not surprising when considering the high dropout rates and dissatisfaction of patients with PTSD who are only prescribed conventional medicine intervention such as CPT, PE, and/or an array of medications, but no CAM.

Therefore, it is essential to continue to conduct empirically-based studies that focus on these high dropout rates and patient dissatisfaction. Research needs to focus on studying and evaluating the efficacy of complementary medicine such as meditation to be added to a patient's treatment plan. A complementary treatment intervention offers a more holistic approach to treatment choices for patients with PTSD.

Health maintenance organizations have become aware of the dissatisfaction and the high dropout rates among patients, and are aware of the market (clients) to which they need to offer CAM treatment options.

A reaction to the dissatisfaction, the Department of Defense, VA, and some health insurance carriers such as Tricare are currently offering coverage for acupuncture or chiropractic work to their members. Also, the transcendental meditation organization working with the David Lynch Foundation are now offering grants and discounted prices to potential students and service members of the armed forces to learn the transcendental meditation technique if they can bring a prescription letter from a health care provider they have seen, (i.e., LCSW, PsyD, PhD, or MD; Dillbecie, 1977, 1987)

The National Institute of Health (2013) identified the percentage of Americans who use CAM is 38%, according to a National Health Interview Survey of 2007 (Meditation programs for stress and wellbeing, 2013). For any health maintenance organization to survive, it is going to need to embrace the future of health care and offer to members coverage for complementary treatments to conventional treatments. This will not only help them to maintain their current subscribers, but will help them garner a larger share of the health care insurance market (National Institute of Health, 2013). Based on the patient dissatisfaction cited by National Institute of Health (2013) and the high dropout rates of allopathic medicine, meditation needs to be seriously considered as another complementary treatment intervention, and continual studies need to be conducted on its efficacy for a whole array of health issues.

Meditation-An Overview

The conceptual framework of meditation is simply a sociocultural response to a changing worldview. The change in attitude about how to reduce anxiety across the globe that is occurring now alongside the rapid strides in science and technology, and the inevitable increases in natural disasters the world is seeing through climate change, wars, and the ever-growing communal hatred among different groups within society is driving the need for change (Maharishi Mahesh Yogi, 1999). The practice of meditation is designed to bring into being a shift in one's consciousness, to move away from an active outward-oriented focus, and employ a direct process toward a receptive and tranquil approach with a move from an external focus of attention to an internal one (Maharishi Mahesh Yogi, 1995).

Borman, Golshan, Thorp, Wetherell, and Lang (2009) highlighted that a meditation practice can help to create a deeper sensitivity to perceptual and cognitive stimuli. The practice can also help to facilitate a change in a person's awareness and reaction to themselves, to others, and their own environment.

A meditation program and its focus are to separate one's self for a brief time from the course of daily life, and to turn off the active mode of normal consciousness to enable one to enter a complementary mode. In meditative exercises, normal consciousness is a personal construction, and it can be extended to a new mode of operation, the complementary mode (Maharishi Mahesh Yogi, 1995). Brauser (2011) discussed that for patients who work through the pain of PTSD, it is neither a peaceful nor a pleasant process and, at times, the patient may choose to deal with his or her pain by avoiding or repressing the negative aspects of their mind.

Lord (2010) had a discourse regarding the value of having a meditative dialog, how important this process can be, and how it can offer a simple way to cultivate what the author calls "sacred space in psychotherapy and in one's life" (Lord, 2010, p. 270). Lord expounded on how the use of a meditative dialog can create a "sacred space," and can be accessed as the therapist and the client engage collaboratively in the quest for transformation through psychotherapy (2010, p. 269).

Meditation as a complementary treatment intervention

The practice of meditation helps a person to learn how to live and how to tune in to his or her body (Lord, 2010, p. 272). Rees (2011) identified meditation as an efficacious intervention method of treatment that can help to reduce, and or possibly eliminate, the symptoms of PTSD anxiety and hypertension, (Saris et al., 2012). As a process, it can be dynamic, and it can help facilitate an individual to change his or her paradigm on how he or she perceives the world (Maharishi Mahesh Yogi, 1999).

Lord (2010) posited that using a meditative dialog can help to improve the ways an individual manages stress in a positive and focused process with clarity. Stress permeates the world, and it alone can be a major precipitating factor that can contribute to the creation of a negative environment, an environment that ultimately affects the overall emotional and physical health of all people in society (Maharishi Mahesh Yogi, 1999). Sayers, Farrow, Ross, and Oslin (2009) identified the rates of family readjustment problems of recent Iraq or Afghanistan conflict veterans screened in primary care, and who were referred for psychiatric evaluation. Sayers et al. (2009) also sought to determine whether the prevalence of these problems was greater for those with psychiatric diagnoses and substance abuse problems, compared to those without these conditions.

The military service members studied by Sayers et al. (2009) frequently choose ways to deal with their stress other than through the accepted western traditional forms of medicine (i.e., allopathic) that can have many undesirable side effects. Subsequently, these forms of treatment (i.e., traditional) are often avoided by patients seeking help with their anxiety because of these negative side effects.

When life and death were their constant companions and their combat experiences are loaded into the neuro network of their brain, a veteran who has been in combat for long periods has difficulty adjusting to a normal life (Seahorn & Seahorn, 2008, p. 136). The stress in the world has helped to lead to an increase in aggression and an escalation of violence all over the world (Maharishi Mahesh Yogi, 1999).

In the book, Maharishi Mahesh Yogi (1999) believed that stressors have helped to create an incessant expansion of anxiety levels in society for quite a while, and the newspapers often are covered with stories of crime, wars, bullying, and other assaults to indicate that the anxiety levels have been rising exponentially. The current state of stress presents an opportunity for researchers to conduct studies and evaluations to determine whether the practice of meditation can be an effective complementary therapy and whether it can be considered a complementary treatment intervention with allopathic western medicine to treat anxiety.

The premise of meditation posits that external conditions cannot be altered, but one can change how one perceives them. The practice of meditation can be useful to reduce or eliminate the effects of stress on a person's life, and to bring change within one's self and in one's own perspective on how one sees issues in one's own life (Maharishi Mahesh Yogi, 1999). The practice of meditation can contribute to the lowering of anxiety symptoms, and can help to improve an individual's focus. The improvement of one's ability to retain new information can help an individual to stay focused (Horowitz, 2010). The literature review examines studies that specifically deal with the efficacy of meditation as a complementary treatment intervention for veterans and others with PTSD. There also is a discussion of how various meditation practices (techniques) compare to other treatments in treating PTSD symptoms; and to what degree, if any, does the practice of meditation offer a complementary treatment intervention that can help reduce PTSD symptoms in veterans and others.

There is an examination of the theoretical and empirical basis for meditation as a treatment intervention for PTSD. Furthermore, which one of the three meditation technique(s) shows the most promise in reducing PTSD anxiety symptoms? Fundamental to all meditation techniques is the cultivation of mental focus, and the way in which it is directed differentiates the meditation techniques practiced (Lang et al., 2012).

Comparison and contrast of the three meditation techniques

Lang et al. (2012) reviewed 118 articles from 1985-2012 with empirically supported treatments for PTSD to determine if there was a good theoretical and empirical basis for each of the three types of meditation techniques (open, focused, and transcendent meditation) as a complementary treatment for patients suffering from PTSD symptoms. The review was comprehensive, and it was a side-by-side comparison and contrast of the mechanism and applicability to PTSD. It presented empirical support for the three different meditation techniques (Travis & Shear, 2010).

Lang et al. (2012) proposed that mindfulness (i.e., open) meditation had the best empirical support for the treatment of PTSD, but the mantra/mantrum (i.e., transcendent meditation) technique showed the most promise. They also established that the compassion (i.e., focused meditation) technique had not been evaluated for anxiety disorders, but it could possibly complement exposure-based therapy and cognitive therapy.

Goldin, Wiveka, and Gross (2009) focused on social anxiety disorder. It is a common and frequently debilitating condition, and is characterized by an intense fear of evaluation in social or performance situations. The symptom of fear in social anxiety disorder correlates with the fear of being around others in a crowd comparable to someone who is suffering from PTSD. Murata et al. (2004) focused on Zen meditation, which is considered a focused meditation technique because its emphasis is on sustained attention and breath control. I also reviewed trait anxiety levels, and evaluated the broad array of accepted empirically-founded psychometric instruments used to measure anxiety of the participants who were undergraduate students practicing the Zen meditation technique in this outstanding study (Myers & Young, 2012).

Trait anxiety can differ according to how individuals have conditioned themselves to respond to and manage their stress (Murata et al., 2004). What may cause anxiety and stress in one person may not generate any emotion in another individual. People can react to the same situation differently based on their perception of what they witness.

An individual who has a high level of trait anxiety is often quite easily stressed and anxious (Murata et al., 2004). Murata et al. (2004) identified that trait anxiety is a state of heightened emotions that develop in response to danger or fear of a particular situation. Anderson et al. (1999) also determined that trait anxiety can contribute to a degree of physical and mental paralysis, preventing performance of a task, or where performance is severely affected (Eppley & Abrams, 1989). Someone who has a lower trait anxiety level is able to meditate quicker with a predominance of internalized attention over relaxation, versus someone who has a higher trait anxiety level with a predominance of relaxation over internalized attention (Murata et al., 2004).

The focused meditation technique reviewed by Murata et al. (2004) would not be an effective meditation technique to treat PTSD trauma survivors. Like PE, the practice of focused meditation by a patient suffering from PTSD symptoms or a high level of trait anxiety could easily trigger arousal, re-experiencing symptoms, and possibly avoidance. The mechanism of focused meditation is to internalize attention, and patients with lower anxiety levels can more readily induce focused meditation with a predominance of internalized attention, not patients who have higher levels of anxiety.

The discussion by Goldin et al. (2009) on social anxiety disorder and Murata et al. (2004) regarding trait anxiety illustrates the similarities of the symptoms of social anxiety disorder, trait anxiety, and PTSD. The symptoms are frequently debilitating and are characterized by an intense fear of evaluation in social or performance situations, and there is a conscious act of being avoidant around others in a crowd; this often includes their own family and friends.

Trauma survivors often feel very anxious and fearful, and often have trouble falling or staying asleep. They experience irritability or outbursts of anger and have significant problems concentrating or focusing on tasks as discussed in Clement (2005). In the arousal symptoms of PTSD, they often:

- have difficulty concentrating,
- have exaggerated watchfulness and wariness,

- have irritability or outbursts of anger,

- have difficulty falling or staying asleep, or

- are easily startled (Everly & Lating, 2002; First, 2002).

Trauma survivors commonly continue re-experiencing or reliving their traumas through a number of symptoms:

- having upsetting memories such as images, thoughts, and perceptions about the trauma;

- experiencing bad dreams and nightmares about the event;

- feeling as if the trauma were happening again (*flashbacks*);

- getting emotionally upset when reminded of the trauma (by something the person sees, hears, feels, smells, or tastes);

- reacting physically (e.g., sweating, heart racing, trouble breathing) when reminded of the trauma (First, 2002).

There are ways for the sufferer to avoid symptoms of PTSD by avoiding thoughts, feelings, and sensations associated with the trauma that can include:

- avoiding trauma-related conversations and

- avoiding places, activities, or people that might be reminders of the trauma (First, 2002).

Symptoms of PTSD include:

- trouble remembering important parts of what happened during the trauma;

- losing interest or not participating in things that one previously enjoyed doing;

- feeling detached or cut off from other people;

- shutting down emotionally or feeling emotionally numb (e.g., trouble having loving feelings for one's family and close friends);

- Feeling as if one's future will be cut short (First, 2002).

Therefore, the use of the focused meditation technique would not be a good recommendation for a patient suffering from PTSD or any other anxiety disorder. Even though the focused meditation technique in these two studies (Goldin et al., 2009; Murata et al., 2004) shows promising results by inducing relaxation, which many PTSD patients can benefit from, there is a potential weakness. The weakness of the technique in treating PTSD or other anxiety disorders is that it focuses on breath and counting. This process could help to open the door to trigger negative intrusive thoughts and memories of trauma. This could possibly harm the patient and others around him or her. Prolonged exposure and cognitive behavioral therapy need to be completed in a controlled clinical setting by a clinician who is qualified to conduct this modality of treatment.

Cloitre et al. (2011) found that two debilitating components of the arousal symptoms of PTSD were feeling agitated and continually on the lookout for danger (i.e., hyper-vigilant) because an individual can experience a torrent of negative and intrusive thoughts. The clinician must have appropriate controls in place to ensure that the patient is provided good medical care, and ensure that the patient is not subjected to a re-experiencing of trauma that can make him or her sensitized again (Cloitre et al., 2011). There is no evidence in the literature review with reference to the focused meditation technique that there has been any clinical oversight, and/ or controls put in place to accommodate this potential outcome by a patient who could become sensitized again through this meditation technique. This needs to be taken into consideration before considering it as a possible complementary treatment for PTSD.

Cahn, Deforme, and Polich (2010) looked at another variation on the focused meditation technique called vipassana. It is similar to Zen meditation because it is also focused. It makes one aware of sensations through the body such as the breath counting in Zen meditation (Simpkins & Simpkins, 2011). Furthermore, the enhancement and awareness of external and internal stimuli could trigger any or all of the three clusters of symptoms of PTSD, and cause great distress to the patient suffering from PTSD (Chiesa, 2010)

The aforementioned caution that Cahn et al., (2010) discussed the use of focused meditation to treat PTSD patients without having good clinical controls to ensure safety, and this concern was amplified in the Libby et al. (2011) review. Both studies recommended that if complementary therapies are to be used then "researchers need to develop treatment protocols that are 'trauma sensitive' for example by emphasizing a sense of safety, predictability, and control" (Libby et al., 2011, p. 7).

Wang et al. (2005, as cited in Libby et al., 2011) established that complementary therapy could prevent or ameliorate the acute increases in distress that could be brought about by exposure-based PTSD treatments, and that 12.6% of individuals with PTSD reported using complementary medicine in the past year. In contrast, this figure from 2005 underestimates the true prevalence of complementary medicine use among individuals with PTSD, as these numbers have dramatically increased over the past five to eight years (National Institute of Health, 2013).

Lang et al. (2012) echoed the concern that there have not been any empirical evaluations/ studies conducted on how effective the focused meditation technique is in treating anxiety disorders. However, the use of it could be a complement to PE and CPT, but only if it is used in a controlled clinical environment. The practice of the focused technique has shown to induce a positive emotional outcome for individuals, and could be used as a complementary treatment intervention with these two evidence-based treatment approaches because of its focus on relaxation (Lang et al., 2012).

The mindfulness (open meditation) technique helps to increase one's self-esteem and helps to decrease an individual's anxiety level. Lochner et al., 2003, Rapee, 1995, Schneier et al., 1994 (as cited in Goldin et al., 2009) stated that seasonal affective disorder can create significant distress and functional impairment in both work and social domains. This is similar to what happens to patients who are struggling with the impairment and disability of their own symptoms when diagnosed with PTSD.

Vujanovic, Niles, Pietrefesa, Schnertz, and Potter (2011) examined how the mindfulness (open meditation) technique could be applied to trauma-related mental health struggles among military veterans. As cited earlier in the discussion, Lang et al. (2012) posited that the mindfulness (open) meditation technique had the best empirical support for the treatment of PTSD. The study examined the integration of mindfulness with current empirically supported treatments for PTSD such as CPT and PE.

The philosophy of mindfulness is to "bring an attitude of curiosity and compassion to the present experience" (Vujanovic et al., 2011, p. 1). One of the positive effects of mindfulness meditation practice on PTSD symptoms is how it helps to enhance emotion regulation and decrease anxiety in an individual (Sears & Kraus, 2009; Toneatto & Nguyen, 2007).

In contrast to the Lang et al. (2012) study, Follette and Vijay (2009, as cited in Vujanovic et al., 2011) stated that the potential clinical utility of integrating mindfulness-based exercises has not been subjected to empirical scrutiny. However, the theoretical and empirical literature suggest that mindfulness meditation practice may serve at least four clinically meaningful functions, and is worth consideration as an effective complementary intervention to treat PTSD symptoms and the benefits of mindful (open) meditation practice (Chiesa & Serretti (2010).

The four benefits of mindful meditation practice are:

1. Regular practice can enhance or create greater present-centered awareness and non-judgmental acceptance of distressing internal states as well as trauma-related triggers.

- If one is more aware of present experience, then he or she is better able to engage effectively in various forms of treatment.

- Regular mindfulness meditation practice has been shown to decrease physiological arousal and stress reactivity.

- Mindful distraction exercises can be used to foster psychological flexibility (Vujanovic et al., 2011, pp. 26-27).

Can the practice of the mindful meditation technique be used as a complementary treatment intervention with the other empirically-based treatment protocols that are trauma sensitive, and can it be efficacious in treating the three clusters of PTSD symptoms with good clinical controls? The answer is a resounding yes if a patient can be taught to manage his or her re-experiencing of PTSD avoidance and arousal symptoms. Mindfulness meditation could make patients more adept and skilled in developing a present-centered awareness. This awareness could help to reduce arousal and stress reactivity, and foster greater psychological litheness (Vujanovic et al., 2011).

Goldin et al. (2009) also examined the effects of the mindfulness (open meditation) technique on patients who were suffering from seasonal affective disorder. Bishop (2002, as cited in Goldin et al., 2009) found that mindful meditation was an effective intervention in reducing the symptoms of social anxiety, depression, rumination, and state anxiety across a wide range of clinical populations. Goldin et al., (2009) hypothesized that the practice of mindfulness meditation could help an individual move from cognitive distortions of the social self toward a more adaptive (i.e. less distorted) mode of his or her own self-referential processing. It is because of this move that there is often a reduction in symptoms. Goldin et al. (2009) had a discourse on the importance of how an individual's self-referential processing is affected, and how this processing helps to contribute to a reduction in self-rumination, and an increase in self-esteem.

Zinn et al. (1992) also assessed the efficacy of the practice of the mindful (open meditation) technique on anxiety. In this study, the participants were diagnosed with generalized anxiety or panic disorder with or without agoraphobia. The study reviewed the effects of the practice of mindfulness meditation, and it was designed to determine the effects of a group stress reduction program on anxiety.

The work of Zinn et al. (1992) was comparable to Goldin et al. (2009) because their participants were composed of non-veterans. There were significant reductions in depression, anxiety, and panic disorder after the completion of the stress reduction and relaxation program they implemented. The formal structure of their programs was similar to Anderson et al. (1999) because the participants also were led by instructors who were trained in the mindfulness (open meditation) technique before they implemented it with patients. In contrast to Anderson et al. (1999), where the classes were only five weeks, the classes were eight weeks in length and were non-veterans in the Zinn et al. (1992) study.

Similar to other techniques of meditation practice such as transcendental meditation (the transcendent technique), the mindfulness (open meditation) technique helps one cultivate greater concentration and relaxation. This is in contrast to the transcendental meditation (transcendent meditation) technique because it trains individuals to attend to a wide range of changing objects of attention while maintaining moment-to-moment awareness (mindfulness), rather that restricting one's focus to a single object such as a mantra/mantram as is used in transcendent meditation (Zinn et al., 1992). The patients who are able to "identify anxious thoughts as thoughts, rather than as 'reality' reported that this alone helped to reduce their anxiety, and increased their ability to encounter anxiety-producing situations more effectively" (Zinn et al., 1992, p. 937).

As cited by Lang et al. (2012), Murata et al. (2004), and Goldin et al. (2009), there have been numerous empirical studies completed concerning focused attention meditation techniques and open monitoring meditation techniques. There have been over 600 studies, just on the transcendental meditation technique alone, that have identified and validated the benefits of this meditation practice technique in many areas of life (Rosenthal, 2011). Transcendent meditation is not a religious practice, but there is a spiritual dimension to it that may lead to results that are more positive, as other studies have concluded (Rosenthal, 2011). Wachholtz and Pargament (2005, 2008) addressed the four research questions that were put forward earlier in Chapter One: (a) Does meditation help in treating PTSD/anxiety symptoms? (b) Does it help in decreasing PTSD symptoms/anxiety? (c) Does meditation contribute to an increase in positive physiological health, and (d) Of the three meditation techniques reviewed, open, focused, and transcendent, which technique is shown to be the most effective in reducing PTSD/anxiety symptoms in veterans and other populations?

Wachholtz and Pargament (2005, 2008) recognized that there was considerable confirmation from a meta-analysis conducted by Alexander et al., 1991, (as cited in Wachholtz & Pargament, 2005) that the transcendent meditation technique had been shown to contribute to a reduction in one's heart rate. It also helped to lower blood pressure, improve one's mental health, and was often more effective than secular meditation techniques that did not have a spiritual component to them. It also helped with the self-regulation of symptoms.

Borman, Liu, and Thorp (2011) found that another variation-mantram (i.e., repeating a sacred word or phrase), which is another facet of the transcendent meditation technique, helped to reduce the severity of PTSD symptoms in veterans with military trauma. This is similar to a mantra, which is also a component of the transcendent meditation technique.

It is essential to discuss the difference between the mantram and the mantra. Whenever people use a mantram, they are only saying a sacred word or phrase that they have chosen, and they are saying it as often as they want to, or when they need to during the day to help them deal with their stress. (Borman, Golshan, Thorp, Wetherell, & Lang, 2009; Borman et al., 2011). However, when someone uses the mantra variation that Maharishi Mahesh Yogi brought to the West, which is what is known now as the transcendent meditation technique, he or she needs to sit comfortably with his or her eyes closed for 15-20 minutes twice daily while mentally experiencing a meaningless sound, termed a mantra, which is given by the teacher of transcendental meditation to the practitioner (Maharishi Mahesh Yogi, 1995).

Both of these variations discussed in Borman et al. (2009, 2011) regarding mantram (i.e., saying a sacred word) and the mantra (i.e., mentally experiencing a meaningless sound) as discussed by Maharishi Mahesh Yogi (1995) have proven to be effective in reducing anxiety and PTSD symptoms (Lang et al., 2012). The focus of Wacholtz and Pargament (2005, 2008) addressed the important question of whether meditation with a spiritual component is a critical ingredient of meditation practice. They also looked at how effective is it versus secular meditation, and if the use of relaxation techniques by patients has an effect on a patient's spiritual, psychological, cardiac, and pain outcomes.

Stewart and Lipton, 2002 (as cited in Wacholtz & Pargament, 2008) established that individuals who suffered from migraine headaches often suffer because of high levels of anxiety and a poor quality of life. They further found that through the practice of spiritual meditation such as the transcendent technique, sufferers of migraine headaches reported a positive effect on positive emotional and physical health. Accordingly, they also acknowledged in the re-experiencing symptom cluster of PTSD that a patient often reacted physically, often manifesting into physiological distress (e.g., sweating, heart racing, trouble breathing, and pounding head that often results in a migraine headache) when reminded of the trauma.

Borman et al. (2011) wanted to determine if a person's spiritual wellbeing could mediate PTSD changes in veterans with military-related PTSD, and if an increase in a person's existential, spiritual wellbeing actually mediates reductions in self-reported PTSD symptoms. They also wanted to determine if these reductions in symptoms were directly correlated with a group mantram intervention. Their study used the mantram (transcendent meditation) technique with their participants such as those in Wacholtz and Pargament (2008) and Borman et al. (2005, 2009). In all of these studies, significant findings supported their hypotheses.

Alexander et al. (1991, as cited in Wachholtz & Pargament, 2005) addressed that meditation can suppress stress reactions and even reverse some of the negative consequences caused by prolonged exposure to stressors such as chronic pain or trauma.

Maharishi Mahesh Yogi believed that the spiritual nature of TM shifts the mind away from physical and mundane concerns to a focus on the larger universe and the individual's place within it, and this focus leads to spiritual awareness (Maharishi Mahesh Yogi, 1995).

Borman et al. (2009) and Anderson et al. (1999) have a comparable premise to Lang et al. (2012). All of them have successfully related the fact that positive outcomes come from the practice of meditation with different populations, and the practice of it has shown to reduce an individual's stress and anxiety levels.

Anderson et al. (1999) posited that meditation could have a positive impact on the perceived stress level in teachers. Their study was unique because it looked at perceived stress levels in teachers and presented findings that are promising for the practice of transcendent meditation. It contributed to a significant reduction in their perceived stress levels in a highly stressed occupation.

Lang et al. (2012) postulated from their review that meditation also was effective in treating anxiety. They conducted an in-depth analysis of all three meditation techniques discussed in Chapter One. They conducted a thorough and comprehensive examination in their extensive literature review on the efficacy of meditation.

Their findings also support and validate a similar hypothesis put forth by Borman et al., (2005, 2009) and Anderson et al. (1999). Moreover, the outcomes answer the four research questions advanced in this study: How does meditation practice (technique) compare to other methods of treating PTSD symptoms, and to what degree if any, does meditation practice (technique) complement treatment intervention in reducing PTSD symptoms in veterans or others?

The studies reviewed by Kroesen et al., (2002) have presented numerous positive emotional and physical health effects that have been reported because of practicing one of the three meditation techniques presented in this study.

Borman et al. (2005, 2009, 2011), Anderson et al. (1999), Lang et al. (2012), and Goldin et al. (2009) also substantiated Kroesen et al. (2002). All of them cited the numerous positive emotional and physical health outcomes that have been reported from patients who practice meditation. These studies have covered an array of dissimilar populations the members of which were suffering from stress and anxiety, and all wanted to find an intervention that could address their symptoms.

Stewart and Lipton, 2002 (as cited in Wacholtz & Pargament, 2008) ascertained that individuals who suffered from migraine headaches did so as a result of having high levels of anxiety and a poor quality of life. They cited that spiritual meditation practices such as the transcendent technique as a CAM were helpful in creating a positive effect on emotional and physical health, and, accordingly, could help aid in reducing migraine headaches.

Wachholtz and Pargament et al. (2005) also showed that patients who practiced the spiritual (transcendent meditation) technique had demonstrated greater pain tolerance. They affirmed that an increased pain tolerance level contributed to an improvement in overall emotional and physical health of these patients. The espousal of the relevance of CAM among health care providers, and the efficacy of using meditation as a treatment modality, are supported by what McLay et al. (2013) stated in definition number two of CAM; it does not fit within the conventional medicine conceptualization, but it does not directly challenge it either. It can serve as a complementary to conventional medicine.

Borman et al. (2009) highlighted that a major debilitating symptom for PTSD sufferers is insomnia. They established that if a patient repeats his or her mantram (spiritual meditation technique) while falling asleep at night, then this technique helped to aid the patient with PTSD to manage his or her sleep issues more effectively.

The assumption presented by Borman et al. (2009) was that the positive outcome with enhanced sleep might be an outcome of the strengthening of the mind-body connection between the mantram and the body's relaxation, with the continual mantram while falling asleep. The researchers in this study recognized and deduced that the connection and technique were contributing factors to the positive outcome of improved sleep with longer intervals of time before being awakened by nightmares.

Halligan, Michael, Wilhelm, Clark, and Ehlers (2006) observed the heart rate response to the voluntary recall of trauma memories in an effort to determine if there was a connection or any relationship to PTSD. Another physical symptom that is reported by patients who are diagnosed with PTSD is high blood pressure; if left untreated, it can become detrimental to an individual's cardiovascular system. The importance of this study was to determine if there is a direct correlation with high blood pressure and voluntary recall by a patient.

The process of recall and taking a patient through the trauma are part of the foundation of CPT and PE, which are approved and accepted treatment interventions in health care treatment settings. Halligan et al. (2006) found that there was evidence of considerable enhanced physiological reactivity to trauma cues that were correlated with PTSD. Likewise, trauma survivors have shown higher heart rates and higher blood pressure numbers when exposed through trauma reminders (cues) than trauma survivors without PTSD (Bernardi et al., 2001)

Foa and Kozak (1986, as cited in Halligan et al., 2006) found that the degree of physical activation, such as an increase in blood pressure or increase in heart rate, was directly related to intentional trauma recall, which is the cornerstone of PE.

Wachholtz and Pargament (2005) discovered that the transcendent meditation technique reduced blood pressure, and it did not have the negative side effects of drowsiness, fatigue, or being unable to function that are often reported by PTSD patients. The aforementioned side effect symptoms are often associated with conventional medication management used today to control blood pressure. Medications may be effective in reducing blood pressure in patients but, sometimes, the side effects make the patient unable to function in his or her daily activities.   Brauser (2011) advanced that meditation may alleviate PTSD symptoms, and can be an effective intervention that can be tolerated with no adverse side effects, and could be used as an effective complementary treatment intervention with conventional medical treatment such as CPT, PE, or pharmacotherapy for patients diagnosed with this complex and challenging disorder to treat (McAllister, 2009).

Meditation seems to have a broad range of applications with positive outcomes throughout different clinical populations and health concerns other than just veterans suffering from PTSD anxiety (Grosswald & Yellin, 2011; Horowitz, 2010; Rees, 2011; Rosenthal, 2011; Shapiro, Walsh & Briton, 2003).

Borman et al. (2009) made conjecture that meditation combined with treatment as usual, (i.e., medication and case management alone) could be a very effective complementary therapy to treat, and/or reduce, chronic PTSD symptoms in veterans.

Borman et al. (2009) evaluated the efficacy of a portable, private meditation-based mantram-sacred word (i.e., the transcendent meditation technique), and sought to determine if the technique was effective for veterans with chronic PTSD. They wanted to determine if the meditation repetition program they were using was an effective addition to the treatment as usual (TAU) program they were using for treating and reducing chronic PTSD symptoms in veterans.

The Anderson et al. (1999) study design was to assess the effectiveness of a standardized mantra (transcendent meditation technique) in treating 91 teachers with perceived stress or anxiety. Both Borman et al. (2009) and Anderson et al. (1999) employed a formalized method of teaching the meditation technique to their participants. The subjects in these studies reported a symptom reduction with anxiety.

Borman et al. (2009) postulated that with the addition of the variable of a mantra repetition program and the TAU program, it could help to reduce PTSD symptoms as opposed to just the TAU, which only included medication and case management. In contrast to Borman et al. (2009), where the veterans used a mantram repetition daily and were instructed to track it; in Anderson et al. (1999), the teachers were instructed to use the standard mantra meditation technique twice per day for 20 minutes, both at school and at home, which were both part of the transcendent technique of meditation.

Anderson et al. (1999) presented a discourse on the alarming percentage of teachers (>50%) leaving the profession in their first five years, and teaching being identified as one of the three most stressful professions by several insurance companies. Some insurance companies have placed teachers into a high-risk group for various types of insurance coverage, (e.g. health and life).

Lang et al. (2012) discussed the millions of people each year who are exposed to traumatic events. Even though teachers are not exposed to combat-related trauma on a battlefield, they are often exposed to a continual battle zone when they often work in schools that are located in neighborhoods with high crime rates, and where drive-by shootings and gang attacks are an everyday occurrence that only exacerbates the anxious perception they have about their profession.

Summary

Combat stress in war is as old as man and combat, and it is very comparable to combat stress in many crime-ridden neighborhoods. Combat stress was finally added in 1980 to the *American Psychological Association Diagnostic Statistical Manual* as PTSD. In assessing stress and even the perception of stress, it is important to continually evaluate the effects that it has on veterans, teachers, students, and others who are suffering from anxiety. Conducting continual evaluations and analyses that indicate positive outcomes can help to continue to raise awareness regarding the efficacy of meditation among health care workers as a complementary medical intervention to treat anxiety successfully.

A safe and healthy emotional reintegration into society for a soldier is important for them to assimilate back into society, and to reintegrate back with their families. It is also important for a student to be able to experience a healthy learning environment in a safe school. A school has a universal philosophy that states learning needs to occur in a safe and stress-free zone, and teachers need to be free of anxious thoughts (Anderson et al., 1999).

In a significant study that adds to a growing repertoire of additional and respected empirical research concerning stress and anxiety, Anderson et al. (1999) focused on measuring and assessing perceived occupational stress levels in teachers. There will undoubtedly be increases in health care costs that will be due to the effects of chronic stress, and this will often lead to many other complex and serious health problems. These health problems will contribute to an increase in the number of sick days taken, and they will have an enormous effect on learning because the learning continuum is interrupted for students (Anderson et al., 1999).

The stigma of being diagnosed with PTSD/anxiety can be terrifying for anyone. It can provoke numerous negative feelings that have a direct and negative effect on an individual's personal and professional relationships (Pietrzak, Johnson, Goldstein, Malley, & Southwick, 2009). The good news is there are some veterans who are choosing to take a more active role in their health care than the veterans of yesterday's wars (Kroesen et al., 2007; National Institute of Health, 2013).

The veterans are doing their own research by conducting searches on Google, asking questions of their health care providers, and through monitoring of their own conventional health care. Because of easy and accessible information, the veterans of today's recent wars appear to be better informed than the veterans prior to the OEF/OIF/OND wars.

They are pursuing more holistic approaches to CAM, and are requesting their conventional health care providers, and the Veterans Administration (VA) health care centers to be knowledgeable about CAM, and to offer it in conjunction with other accepted evidence-based treatments available to them (Brauser, 2011).

Earlier, I discussed the problem with high dropout rates and the dissatisfaction among countless veterans and others who are suffering from PTSD and a variety of anxiety symptoms. High dropout rates can be a significant barrier to care for these veterans. What can help is an openness and to actively listen to the veterans regarding their health care and what they are really saying about their treatment, and this can be a step in the right direction. The negative feelings that are associated with PTSD can often cause distress in any relationship with others including health care providers (Lang et al., 2012).

The data presented in Lang et al. (2012) indicated that the high dropout rates are related directly to resistance by patients toward empirical-evidence-based treatments for PTSD such as CPT and PE. There is also a concern that patients often effectively are kept in a vacuum when providers are not open to other approaches or are afraid to use them.

The resistance that Lang et al. (2012) cited is due to the discomfort of treatments and the lack of positive outcomes to the various chronic conditions that are reported by many veterans to control pain or reduce intolerable drug side effects. There is over a 20% dropout rate for any exposure-based or cognitive intervention (Lang et al., 2012). A comprehensive review and a comprehensive evaluation of meditation techniques can help to determine if meditation can, in fact, be an effective complementary therapeutic treatment option for veterans, and others diagnosed with PTSD.

Kroesen et al. (2002) provided qualitative data that can help physicians understand how widespread the use of CAM is among their patients and, it is hoped, open their minds to consider a more holistic approach with complementary treatments such as meditation to complement conventional medicine. They need to be open and listen to their patients using active listening skills to determine what a patient is really saying about his or her treatment experiences.

The data from the Kroesen et al. (2002) study can help raise the levels of awareness within the medical community. The awareness can develop insight where the health care providers begin to collaborate more with their patients and develop treatment plans that contain inputs from their patients that include a more holistic approach.

Through the review of numerous studies evaluating meditation as an intervention to treat PTSD symptoms among veterans, there is limited empirical research on this subject. However, this limitation has allowed a narrowing of the scope and focus on the research questions posed in Chapter One. The expanded search in this study produced a comprehensive compilation of reviews and research studies that addressed these concerns. Through the review of all of them, and through the process of identifying themes that addressed the research questions posed, I was able to assemble them into a logical discussion in this literature review.

It was also learned that the practice of meditation, whenever it is used as a complementary treatment, has been effective in reducing anxiety symptoms in other populations. These other populations were struggling with perceived anxiety, PTSD, generalized anxiety, and social anxiety. The expansion and narrowing of the research questions helped to draw effective comparisons and helped to contrast differences between the studies. Hence, the process helped to distinguish and identify effective meditation techniques for veterans and other populations.

As a result of the process, the generalizability of the study was strengthened because of its comprehensive approach to the review of the research that considered not only positive outcomes of emotional health, but also the positive physical outcomes from the practice of meditation. All of the studies reviewed had common themes:

- They were comprised of participants who were dealing with anxiety.
- They used one of the three meditation techniques in their study: open, focused, or transcendent.
- They were comprised of veterans and non-veterans who were dealing with anxiety.

- They all recommended that CAM needs to be evaluated by health care providers, so they are knowledgeable about holistic treatment approaches.

- There needs to be ongoing empirical research on the efficacy of meditation to treat PTSD.

Meditation has been practiced for well over 2500 years as a component of numerous religious traditions and beliefs. The practice of meditation involves an internal effort to self-regulate the mind in some way and is often used to clear the mind, and ease emotional and physical distress (Maharishi Mahesh Yogi, 1995).

In conclusion, there has been limited empirical research on the practice of meditation over the last 10 years, and the sample sizes used have been smaller. There have been some studies that have used inadequate psychometric measuring tools; most of the instruments were self-report survey in the 1970s. The small sample sizes of the earlier studies affected the generalizability of the findings and helped to determine if there were significant findings.

However, the good news is that in the year 2000 there were over 70 studies published in peer-reviewed journals using the terms *mindfulness*, *yoga*, or *meditation*, and in 2011 there were over 560 studies (Grosswald & Yellin, 2011; Horowitz, 2010; Rees, 2011; Rosenthal, 2011; Shapiro, Walsh & Briton, 2003).

The way forward is for awareness to be continually raised among health care providers, and for even more patients to continue to self-advocate for CAM. Change will happen with more health care providers caring about patient dissatisfaction and high dropout rates among their patients receiving solely conventional treatment. This will be a catalyst to help push the health care profession to conduct even more empirical research studies regarding the efficacy of the practice of meditation as an effective complementary treatment intervention for PTSD.

Chapter 3: Research Methods and Procedures

Introduction

The purpose of this study was to determine if meditation, when used as a complementary treatment method, leads to a decrease in PTSD/anxiety symptoms, and to determine which of the three predominant meditation techniques is the most effective in treating PTSD/anxiety.

Of the three most widely used meditation techniques (i.e., open, focused, and transcendent), the transcendent meditation technique will produce the greatest positive impact in treating the psychological and physiological effects of PTSD/and other anxiety disorders.

Research Design

The literature was reviewed to locate, appraise, and synthesize all research on the topic. Choosing the systematic review strengthened all of the research questions because a systematic review, unlike a narrative review, is designed to answer specific clinical questions where several primary studies exist and, thus, it was a good source of clinical evidence for this project. The search and selection criteria for the articles chosen were that all bodies of literature were well defined, and multiple databases were searched. The use of a strict methodology and thoroughness, and the conclusions posited were less biased than a narrative review. The studies reviewed were included primarily based on their adherence to sound scientific methodology.

The literature review was conducted by a comprehensive analysis of more than 120 peer-reviewed studies, articles, documents, and books that had good psychometric measuring tools; were controlled studies; and were generalizable. The next step was to conduct a detailed examination of these studies, which resulted in a subset of 88 studies that focused on trauma and treatment and a further subset of 33 studies that focused specifically on trauma-anxiety and meditation. This process is discussed further in the Data Analysis section of this chapter.

Methodology

There was a comprehensive search performed using Internet resources in the United States and internationally, utilizing the following keywords: (a) PTSD, (b) meditation, (c) veteran, and (d) complementary. The databases were searched from publications from 1977 through to the present (2014). A number of resources were searched, including: CSU Librarian, University Virtual Library, Google Scholar, the American Psychiatric Association website, the National Center for PTSD, VA.gov, the David Lynch Foundation, TM.org, Psych INFO, Medline, NASW, Psych WEB, and other biomedical and social science websites to identify applicable studies.

A review of both alternative and complementary mental health treatment intervention efficacies was conducted. Similarly, only peer-reviewed, empirical research studies, books that represent the results of thousands of clients, or meta-analyses conducted by other researchers that represent the results of hundreds of recent studies involving PTSD/anxiety, meditation, complementarity and/or veterans were considered.

There were also various populations (e.g., teachers, health care workers, veterans, minority students, graduate, undergraduate students, victims of sexual assault, and various nationalities) that were considered. Furthermore, numerous meditation applications in various treatment protocols (in-patient/outpatient patients) also were taken into account in the review (Elder et al., 2008).

There was a screening and narrowing of current meditation techniques, and they eventually were narrowed to three categories (i.e., open, focused, and transcendent). Furthermore, meditation applications for numerous health ailments (e.g., stress, migraines, PTSD, generalized anxiety disorder, panic disorder, and heart disease) were also considered.

Data Analysis

Pre-screening of peer-reviewed studies on the complementary treatment methods for improving overall health using Google Scholar was conducted. This resulted in an initial foundation of over 120 peer-reviewed empirically-based studies, articles, books, and meta-analyses conducted by other researchers that were drawn from for this study. Using the following criteria, the studies used for this research were reduced from 120 to 88 articles, books, and meta-analyses conducted by other researchers based upon the following discriminators: (a) the studies used at least 15 participants, (b) the results were attained through a controlled study using professionally accepted statistical protocols, and (c) they utilized an American Psychiatric Association-approved psychometric instrument(s).

This selection process resulted in 88 studies that focused on the effects of trauma on varying populations and the use of approved allopathic treatment interventions including psychotherapy approaches such as cognitive processing therapy, prolonged exposure therapy, and pharmacological treatments (see Appendix A). Also included in these 88 peer-reviewed studies were 33 that focused specifically on trauma-anxiety and meditation. These 33 studies were used to provide the basis for a comparative analysis of the allopathic treatment methods currently used to treat trauma-anxiety.

There are a limited number of empirically-tested, peer-reviewed studies that examined complementary therapies that were efficacious in treating PTSD, that also conducted empirical data collection and reviewed relevant research concerning the efficacy of meditation in reducing PTSD symptoms that were identified by searching the biomedical and social science databases for primary research material. A search of articles, studies, editorials, book search for studies, and meta-analyses conducted by other researchers that had at least one of the four keywords was conducted. To ensure that relevant studies were not missed, the search terms remained broad: *meditation*, *PTSD*, *veteran*, and *complementary*. No language restrictions were employed. Studies were eligible for consideration in this review if: (a) the focus of the study was meditation, veterans, PTSD, and complementarity and (b) there was at least one of the keywords (Appendix A).

Assumptions

A proper meditation technique involves the education, training, and practice of concentrated focus on a sound, object, visualization, the breath, movement, or attention itself in order to increase awareness of the present moment, reduce stress, and promote relaxation (Lang et al., 2012). The assumption is that in any study in which meditation was used, the study participants were trained in proper effective techniques of meditation.

Although there are studies involving the positive effects that meditation has on everyday individuals, the focus of this study was to study the effects of proper meditation techniques on stress and the physiological effects that stress creates in the body.

Therefore, another assumption is that the presenting problems of individuals who reported trauma and who were identified as having PTSD, social anxiety disorder, trait anxiety, generalized anxiety disorder, or other associated, physical ailments, were substantiated prior to the studies measuring the efficacy of meditation on these symptoms.

Limitations of the Study

The quantitative meta-analysis method other researchers used in their studies that I reviewed helped in analyzing the effects of meditation on a vast segment of different populations affected by stress, anxiety, and trauma. The theoretical study does not allow me to speak directly as the researcher to effect the selection of the population, control measures, or implementation of the intervention.

Another limitation is that there is little evidence concerning any negative effects of meditation. Numerous articles and blogs discuss negative effects of meditation, but there are a limited number of empirically-based studies supporting the negative effects of meditation on an individual. More will be discussed on this topic in the Findings section of Chapter 4.

The diagnosis of PTSD only became acknowledged as a disorder in 1980 by the American Psychiatric Association. Consequently, mental health professionals have only been working with this diagnosis for 34 years as of the time of this writing. Mental health professionals can be slow to embrace complementary techniques if they are not considered part of allopathic medicine. Therefore, the holistic study of PTSD is still in its early stages.

Chapter 4: Findings

Findings

Based on the principles of methodology, sample size, and generalizability, I identified over 100 empirically-based research studies, books, meta-analyses conducted by other researchers, and systematic reviews that were reviewed in this study. Of these more than 100 studies that were reviewed, 33 were in the final selection. This final selection of 33 empirically-based research studies, articles, books, and meta-analyses conducted by other researchers covering the timespan from 1991-2013 utilized over 4,475 participants and answered all of the research questions confirming that meditation is highly effective in the treatment of symptomology associated with PTSD/anxiety as a CAM, and of the three meditation techniques reviewed in this study, TM is the most effective technique of meditation addressing the negative physiological effects of PTSD/anxiety.

Introduction

The purpose of this study was to examine the questions of meditation as a complementary treatment to treat PTSD symptoms, and what, if any, is the most effective form of meditation to reduce PTSD symptoms for this population. How does meditation help in treating PTSD/anxiety symptoms? Is there a decrease in PTSD symptoms/anxiety? Is there an increase in positive physiological health? Moreover, of the three meditation techniques reviewed, open, focused, and transcendent, will the transcendent technique prove to be the most effective in reducing PTSD/anxiety symptoms in veterans or others?

Additionally, the purpose of the study was to create an in-depth discussion of how veterans suffering from PTSD symptoms are currently being treated, and if meditation might be valuable in treating veterans suffering from PTSD. The article by Howard (p.A17, 2013) discussed that the health community was beginning to embrace meditation, and that in order to move forward was to review the current PTSD allopathic interventions and treatment outcomes, and to continue to educate the medical community to embrace complementary alternative medical interventions (Howard, 2013).

Therefore, by discovering through a thorough analysis of the data, a comprehensive evaluation of recent empirical research on open, focused, and transcendent meditations, the goal was to determine if meditation use as a CAM treatment intervention is helpful in treating PTSD symptoms. The discoveries made in this study were organized around the four keywords used to narrow the search (i.e., PTSD, veterans, meditation, and complementary). The conclusions posited by the researchers were qualitative and, therefore, positioned.

This study analyzed 88 studies that focused on the effects of trauma on varying populations, and the use of approved allopathic treatment interventions including psychotherapy approaches such as cognitive processing therapy and prolonged exposure therapy, as well as pharmacological treatments, and CAM.

This chapter is a discussion of the results of empirical research in the field, and an exploration of the correlates between a CAM treatment intervention (meditation) that is effective as a complementary treatment intervention without the side effects present in the CPT, PE, and pharmacological interventions currently being used. Every article reviewed was examined. Studies were excluded if they were not generalizable, if they had fewer than 15 participants, or if meditation, veteran, PTSD/anxiety, or complementary was only a minor variable in the study.

Additionally, if a study reviewed did not contribute important information to this study it was omitted. It was noteworthy to discover through the literature review whether there is a connection between the practice of meditation and the improvement in PTSD symptoms with veterans and others.

There has been over 21 years of research in the field (see Figure 1). Additionally, the findings posit that meditation induces not only positive outcomes of emotional health, but also produces positive physical outcomes from the practice of meditation.

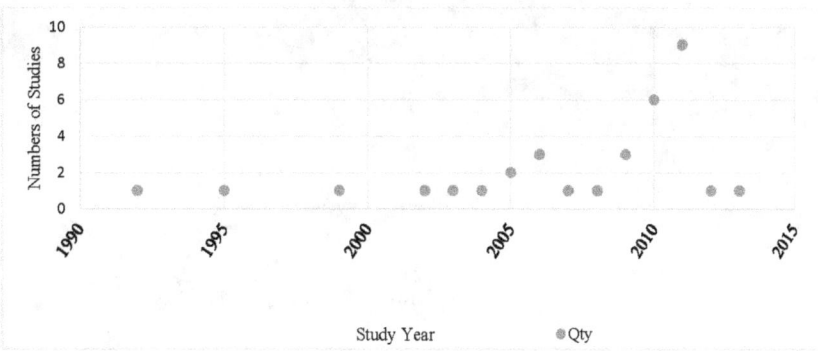

Figure 1. Number of meditation research studies completed by year since 1992.

Note. Figure 1 represents the 21-year span from 1992 to 2013 during which the final studies used for this study were conducted (X-axis = the year the study was completed / Y-axis = the number of studies completed within a particular year.

The practice of meditation is "now widely accepted as a mind-body technique for maintaining holistic health and wellness" (Horowitz, 2010, p. 227). The sample sizes used in the early studies in the 1970s used inadequate psychometric measuring tools; some of them were self-report surveys during this decade. In addition, the small sample sizes of the earlier studies affected the generalizability of the findings and helped to determine if there were significant findings. The studies selected and reviewed were empirical-evidence-based.

Results

It can be concluded that the data supports the conclusions that show that meditation is very effective in helping to reduce anxiety symptoms in not only veteran populations, but other populations as well (see Figure 2). It also can be very helpful to improve emotional regulation for someone suffering from PTSD/anxiety (Newberg, Wintering, Khalsa, Roggenkamp, & Waldman, 2012).

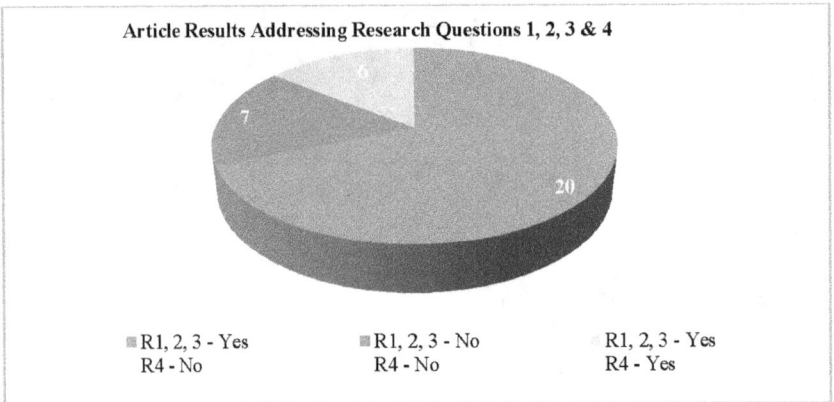

Figure 2. How the data supported the research questions.

Note. Figure 2 represents the breakdown of the final articles, research studies, and meta-analyses conducted by other researchers, books, systematic reviews, and editorials that comprised the final selection used as the basis for this doctoral study concerning whether they addressed research questions one, two, three, and four.

The research findings also indicate that there is a great deal of empirical evidence to support the research questions with very significant positive indicators for effective change that can be useful for clinicians, veterans, and others in making decisions about the best available options for stress reduction among these populations when considering meditation as an effective complementary treatment intervention with allopathic medicine (see Figure 3).

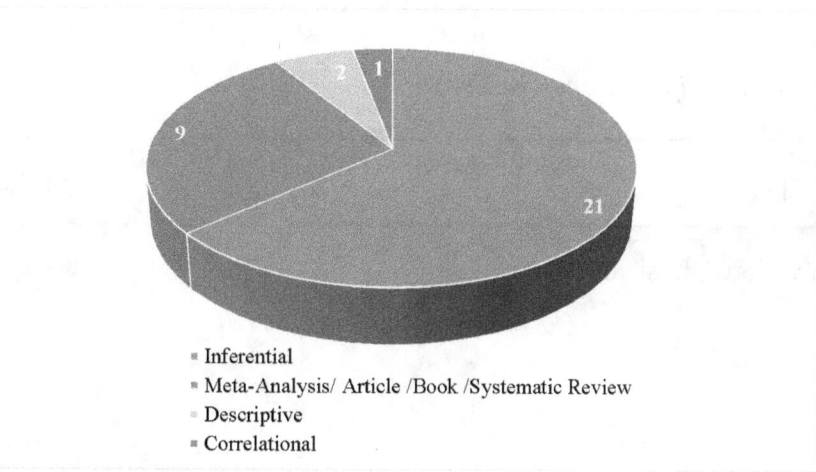

Figure 3. Statistical data analysis.

Note. Chart represents the grouping and data breakdown of all 33 studies by descriptive, inferential, and meta-analysis statistical methods used. Meta-analyses conducted by other researchers were used in this doctoral study to draw some conclusions regarding the efficacy of treating veterans diagnosed with PTSD/anxiety with meditation (see Appendix D).

Populations reviewed other than just the veterans were also struggling with perceived anxiety, PTSD, generalized anxiety, and social anxiety (see Table 2). The expansion and narrowing on the research questions posited helped to draw effective comparisons and to contrast differences. The various populations (e.g., teachers, health care workers, veterans, minority students, graduate, undergraduate students, victims of sexual assault, various nationalities) were all reviewed for this study.

Table 2

Meditation Study Participant Demographics

Participant Type	Participant Count
Clients with various physical/mental issues	1456
Veterans with PTSD	790
Clients diagnosed with PTSD	599
College-age students	505
Youth populations	298
*Other (high school students, teachers, crime victims, and the elderly)	827
Total	4475

Note. Table 2 represents the breakdown of all participants by count and type that were captured in the final articles, research studies, meta-analyses conducted by other researchers, books, systematic reviews, and editorials that comprised the final selection used as the basis for the study in this doctoral study.

In support of research questions one, two, and three, meditation can help someone diagnosed with anxiety because it can help to eliminate the source of stress in the mind and the body, and provide profound relaxation that helps the body to naturally dissolve deeply rooted stresses (Horowitz, 2011). Meditation is a family of practices that train attention and awareness, usually with the objective of fostering psychological and spiritual wellbeing and maturity. It does this by training and bringing one's mental processes under greater voluntary control, and directing them in beneficial ways (Horowitz, 2010).

In support of research questions one, two, and three, there were 14 studies, 6 meta-analyses, 3 systematic reviews, 1 literature review, and one informational article conducted by other researchers, constituting 69% of all studies reviewed. An analysis of the data suggests that meditation is often used by Americans as a complementary medical intervention (Horowitz, 2010, p. 223).

It is currently and generally accepted by many that meditation is a mind-body technique for maintaining holistic health and welfare. According to Horowitz (2010), "meditation has proven to be a safe and effective complementary therapy intervention for treating a variety of conditions because the psychological effects of chronic illness, and pain effects are often not addressed in conventional allopathic treatments" (Horowitz, 2010, p. 227).

The fourth research question focused specifically on exploring three meditation techniques reviewed (i.e., open, focused, and transcendent) to answer this question and to determine, based on all of the studies reviewed and evaluated, whether the transcendent technique is the most effective in reducing PTSD/anxiety symptoms in veterans or others. Six studies (14%) were in support of the fourth research question. Additionally, two studies and two meta-analyses conducted by other researchers supported all four research questions (see Appendix B).

Furthermore, regarding the fourth research question, the discovery through this study clearly indicates that of the interventions used, (a) the mindfulness (focused) meditation technique, (b) progressive muscle relaxation (PMR; open), and (c) the transcendent meditation (TM) technique, the available data support TM as the most effective in virtually all outcomes studied to date (Gaylord, Orme-Johnson, & Travis, 1988; Rausch, Gramling, & Auerbach, 2006; Rees, 2011).

TM has the greater volume of supporting research with the exception of a large volume on mindfulness and more high-quality studies (i.e., prospective randomized controlled design) than the other two approaches. Nearly all of the meta-analyses reviewed by Rees (2011) and other comparative studies show greater effect sizes for the fourth research question. In populations that varied by age, ethnicity, and nationality, TM significantly outperformed PMR in the reduction of high blood pressure among hypertensive patients, conditions for hypertension, anxiety to mortality.

There is compelling evidence regarding the efficacy of TM, which possibly has contributed to lower health care utilization and costs. Rees (2011) proposed that because of this factor, TM is attractive to soldiers, families, and organizations responsible for providing medical and mental health services as the cost to society from combat-related PTSD alone are in the billions of dollars per year and growing. Mindfulness and PMR may have yet undemonstrated beneficial effects on health care costs.

The writings by Maharishi Mahesh Yogi (1995) helped to lay the foundation of what the TM technique is. It is the definitive introduction to the practice of TM. In 8 meta-analysis of 597 studies of over 20,000 subjects, TM significantly outperformed other modalities across a host of outcomes, including improved psychological outcomes and improved health, helps to reverse some of the aging process, lowers high blood pressure, helps to decrease the risk of a stroke, and helps lead to a decreased use of cigarettes, drugs, and alcohol (Rees, 2011).

The TM meditation (transcendent) technique helps to expand the mind to its unlimited cosmic potential (Maharishi Mahesh Yogi, 1995).Only one site was discovered through the research review that was very critical of meditation; it was published by Joe Kellett in June 2010. The website had many negative opinions posted, but there were no scientific or empirical research studies presented to support these negative assertions.

Analysis and Evaluation of Findings

The use of CAM interventions. The 2007 National Health Interview Survey (NHIS) defined what CAM was (National Institute of Health, 2013). The conclusions drawn from the researchers were that the dissatisfaction with medications helped to contribute to the use of CAM. Many of the participants in these studies had begun to move their care beyond the bounds of the conventional allopathic medical system because it was not meeting their needs (National Institute of Health, 2013).

The prevalence of CAM use among individuals was 38%, and for individuals who were using meditation and relaxation it was 17%, with 62.8% of individuals with PTSD using either CAM or traditional mental health services (Libby et al., 2011). It can be suggested that if clinicians did indeed know the use by patients of CAM interventions, then it could possibly help them to maximize benefits for their patients. This knowledge would also help to minimize the risks of both conventional and CAM approaches while providing patient-centered care to individuals with PTSD that have particular mental and physical health care needs. The most common practice of CAM treatment intervention discovered was meditation, and it was discovered that meditation does, in fact, improve one's autonomic regulation, which is in deficit in individuals who are diagnosed with PTSD (Libby et al., 2011).

It was this improvement in autonomic regulation with individuals who had mental health problems that helped them to become the ones who came in seeking meditation, and was among the most frequently cited reasons for seeking help from a complementary provider who could offer to them meditation as a CAM treatment intervention.

It was concluded in the studies reviewed that the combination of conventional and complementary treatment interventions can help to resolve the problematic issues of high dropout rates and dissatisfaction in patients with PTSD that have trouble enduring the conventional western medicine interventions such as medications, CPT, PE, or pharmacology being prescribed (Brauser, 2011).

Studies that did not support Research Questions One, Two, Three, or Four. There were two studies, one meta-analysis conducted by other researchers, and one editorial that did not address the treatment intervention of meditation. However, none of them was able to identify a relationship between the two measured phenomena of research questions one, two, three, and four.

The Sayers et al. (2009) study was not developed with a strong research design, and there was an absence of approved psychometric measuring tools. The absence of appropriate administered psychometric tools, the use of a self-report survey, and the absence of meditation being studied are compelling factors to conclude that this is a meager study (Appendix C1).

Similarly, the Schnurr et al. (2010) editorial also did not support the fourth research question. It only identified cognitive behavioral therapies such as PE, CPT, and EMDR as first-line treatments for PTSD; CAM (or meditation) as an intervention was not considered in the treatment protocols for PTSD.

Additionally, the Hamblen et al. (2010) meta-analysis did not support the four research questions either because of the absence of meditation as a CAM in this study. It was an overview of using psychotherapy for treating PTSD, and they reviewed a variety of cognitive behavioral treatments including psychoeducation, anxiety management, exposure, and cognitive restructuring, but not meditation. This is comparable to the Halligan (2006) study where meditation was not considered as a complementary treatment intervention.

Summary

The in-depth facet of meditation can be found in Chapter Two of this study, and it can be summarized that "meditation has proven to be a safe and effective complementary treatment intervention for treating a variety of conditions because the psychological effects of chronic illness and pain effects are often not addressed in conventional allopathic treatments" (Horowitz, 2010, p. 227).

There are data for healthy psychological correlates with the use of CAM (meditation). Therefore, it can be concluded that cultural perspective and personal interpretation are both decisive measures that influence the stigma and reluctance to embrace CAM by allopathic healthcare providers. It is critical that there is an understanding of the causes of this stigma, and possibly what can be done to make meditation more universally appealing and accepted by mainstream society.

Chapter 5: Conclusion and Discussion

Discussion of Findings

The purpose of this doctoral study was to evaluate and determine if the use of meditation as a complementary treatment intervention with allopathic medicine is efficacious in reducing the negative symptoms associated with PTSD/anxiety and increasing positive physiological outcomes associated with good health (i.e., reduction of hypertension, improved relaxation and mental functioning, and increase in emotional regulation).

My focus was on identifying four keywords proposed for this study, which were (a) complementary, (b) meditation, (c) PTSD/anxiety, and (d) veterans, with the purpose of converging on the most pertinent empirical research available (Posadzki, Parekh, & Glass, 2010). This proved to be an effective process because it helped to identify and narrow the focus on the area of interest and a subsequent study in the study. Studies that lacked good research design controls or that did not use accepted psychometric instruments to measure outcomes were discarded (from 120 to 88 included in the annotated bibliography) as were studies that were not generalizable to those suffering from PTSD/anxiety.

A weighted analysis was then utilized to narrow the selection of studies on which the study focused; this helped to produce the most comprehensive information to address the four research questions in the study. This led to a further reduction of articles from 88 to 33. The selection criteria helped to determine that of the four keywords selected, at least one needed to be mentioned in a study in order to be considered relevant. The studies selected were controlled; they employed appropriate psychometric measuring instruments to measure outcomes, and they were generalizable. All of the studies used for this analysis encompassed over 21 years of research in the field.

The type and count of participants for the final number of studies reviewed for this study varied. The participants were volunteers, and they gave their written consent on forms that described the study's main risk and benefits, and the study's assurance that their confidentiality would be maintained. They were also selected and deemed eligible for the studies by the researchers only if they could participate safely. Finally, the participants of these studies were required to provide complete and correct information to the researcher(s).

The psychometric tests that were used in these studies were structured, and they had standardized assessment procedures, which helped to facilitate the researchers to measure aspects of a client's functioning. The 46 psychometric tools varied in the degree of formality between structured observations, such as questionnaires, to prescribed tasks, which were administered under carefully controlled standardized conditions. These tools were used 77 times in these studies (Appendix C).

These psychometric tools were structured, standardized, and measured cognitive, behavioral, and emotional health. The testing occurred in a structured and controlled environment, and the usage of these tests was consistent with normal professional practice. Last, the researchers selected appropriate psychometric assessment instruments and procedures for the objectives of the assessment (Appendix C).

Hence, the controlled studies provided overwhelming support that there are positive outcomes for the four research questions. The tools were grouped for measuring depression and anxiety for the first three research questions. Accordingly, for the fourth research question, the tools were grouped under this category based upon the amount to which physiological health was measured. The psychometric measuring tools used in these studies enabled the effective measuring of the results of all four research questions, which measured PTSD, anxiety, depression, and physiological health. This also contributed to insight into the ever-increasing health benefits of TM in contrast to open and focused meditation techniques (Appendix C).

After examining over 100 peer-reviewed research studies, journal articles, meta-analyses conducted by other researchers, editorials, books, and literature reviews, there is a strong body of evidence to support the use of meditation to effectively reduce the negative effects of PTSD/ anxiety and increase positive physiological health.

Furthermore, the body of evidence that was reviewed produced findings that indicated that the TM technique was, by far, the most documented and effective form of meditation. The collective body of knowledge used for this literature review was scientifically sound and generalizable to people across a multitude of ages, socioeconomic backgrounds, educational levels, ethnicities, both genders, and varying stages of physical and mental health.

In review of 8 meta-analyses conducted by other researchers, of over 597 studies with over 20,000 subjects, TM had significantly outperformed other modalities across a host of outcomes, including improved psychological outcomes and a decreased use of cigarettes, drugs, and alcohol (Rees, 2011).

Implications and Recommendations

America has now been at war longer than ever in its history as a nation—over 13 years. This newest generation of service members returning home from wars around the globe struggle with trying to put their lives back together, and return to a place of balance and optimal health. In addition to being a highly effective complementary treatment intervention for veterans diagnosed with PTSD/anxiety, studies also clearly indicated that many others could benefit from the positive effects of the practice of TM. Stress and anxiety-related injuries and illnesses are the invisible epidemic of the 21st century throughout the western world. There is no shortage of data that suggests that there are staggering costs to both the workforce and to healthcare because of the ill effects of stress and anxiety.

At a time when Americans are abusing prescription medications at epidemic levels, meditation offers a healthy and highly effective alternative. The conclusion drawn from the researchers was that the dissatisfaction with medications has helped to contribute to the use of CAM. Kroessen (2002) was the first to address CAM use among veterans. There is no reason to believe that meditation would interfere with psychotherapy or pharmacotherapy, but it could facilitate other treatment approaches.

The peer-reviewed research clearly indicates that there are significant physiological and psychological improvements in individuals who are practitioners of meditation across a variety of demographics. These include high school students in China and America, teachers in America, health care workers, undergraduate students, and victims of violent crime, as well as those with numerous physical injuries and illnesses (Horowitz, 2010).

Cloitre (2011) discovered that the majority of treatment providers endorsed as a first- and second-line intervention the need for "emotional regulation interventions," and "anxiety stress management interventions." Likewise, a meditation intervention was frequently identified as a second-line intervention for symptom sets (e.g., affect, dysregulation, and disassociation; Overholser, & Fisher, 2009).

Libby et al. (2011) concluded that if clinicians did know of the use by patients of CAM interventions then it could help them to maximize benefits for their patients. This knowledge would also help to minimize the risks of both conventional and CAM approaches while providing patient-centered care to individuals with PTSD that have particular mental and physical health care needs. The most common practice of CAM treatment intervention used was meditation, and it was discovered that meditation does, in fact, improve one's autonomic regulation, which is a deficit in individuals who are diagnosed with PTSD.

If the effects of meditation are so profound, one might ask why more people are not doing it. In clinical practice over the past 25 years, I have identified numerous clients that could undoubtedly benefit from the effects of TM. However, after the idea is proposed to them, they are often reluctant, and when an attempt is made to explore their reluctance to pursue TM further, many cannot clearly communicate to me why they are reluctant.

Future research is warranted to explore the nature and effects of the stigma associated with TM. There is little to no stigma attached to taking a Valium for anxiety, or an Ambien for sleep, but there is a negative stigma associated with the concept of healing oneself through the practice of meditation as a complementary treatment intervention working with allopathic medicine. The recommendation for future research is that it needs to be directed at understanding the causes of this negative stigma, exploring what can be done to overcome it, and how to make meditation more universally appealing and accepted by society.

Virtually all of the meta-analyses conducted by other researchers and the comparative studies show greater effect sizes for TM in conditions for hypertension and anxiety to mortality in populations varied in age, ethnicity, and nationality. TM significantly outperformed PMR in the reduction of high blood pressure among individuals diagnosed with hypertension.

TM has demonstrated lower health care utilization and costs. This fact may make TM attractive to service members in the armed forces and to families and organizations responsible for providing their medical and mental health services. The cost to society from combat-related PTSD alone is in the billions of dollars per year and growing.

If meditation interventions specifically target PTSD/anxiety symptom clusters, then it may be a beneficial complementary treatment intervention for individuals struggling with residual symptoms. Meditation may not appeal to every individual with PTSD/anxiety, but for those who are interested in complementary and alternative approaches, it would be a welcome addition to our repertoire of empirically-supported treatment approaches (Lang, 2012).

Additionally, further efforts are needed to apply meditation practices in clinical settings in ways that are practical, effective, and meaningful (Horowitz, 2010). As cited in Horowitz (2010) "there needs to be a comparison of different types of meditation, and of meditation with other therapies, an evaluation of long-term effects, and further elucidation of the neurobiological and clinical correlates of the non-pharmacologic modality are warranted" (2010, p. 227).

Furthermore, as discussed in Borman (2005), there needs to be (a) future studies that include using an experimental design with larger sample sizes, and (b) other patient populations need to be targeted for study such as patients with HIV/AIDS, and Alzheimer's caregivers. Future studies need to use larger sample sizes over a longer period, as it can help to examine the long-term effects of TM.

In his systematic review, McLay (2013) discussed the limitations of CAM, and the need for the standardization of CAM interventions to be established. Further, he identified that as of July 2012 there had been over 700 publications using the terms *alternative medicine* and *PTSD*, and 48 of these were randomized controlled studies. It is critical that empirical research continues to review psychotherapeutic research concerning manualization. This review process would help to ensure that treatment fidelity is standardized for both clinical applications and for research.

Conclusion

It is my conclusion that meditation, specifically TM, is the most efficacious as a complementary treatment intervention for veterans diagnosed with PTSD/anxiety, and the practice of TM would greatly benefit these veterans as a complementary treatment intervention for those who are treated by the VA healthcare system throughout our nation. The Department of Veteran Affairs primarily uses evidence-based CPT, PE, and pharmacology to treat PTSD with limited effectiveness.

Meditation is a family of practices that can help someone be more attentive and aware, with the objective of fostering psychological and spiritual wellbeing. Thus, with this new level of awareness and attentiveness there is a maturation that occurs that can contribute in helping to bring one's mental processes under greater voluntary control, and to direct them in positive and beneficial ways. The control that is achieved can be used to help cultivate specific mental qualities such as concentration and calm, and emotions such as joy, love, and compassion. Through this greater awareness and control, a clearer understanding of oneself and one's relationship to the world develops.

As cited in Lang (2012), there are a number of potential benefits with the integration of meditation-based methods. Most practices are taught in a group format, and they can be taught relatively quickly with minimal cost. The approach has no significant side effects, and the practice has shown to be well tolerated by a wide spectrum of individuals. The practice of meditation is widely accepted as a mind-body technique for maintaining holistic health and wellness. It has proven to be a safe and effective complementary treatment intervention for treating a variety of conditions, and the psychological effects of chronic illness and pain-effects that are not often addressed in conventional allopathic treatments (Horowitz, 2010).

Conclusions of the three modalities discussed in this study and the data reviewed support TM as the most efficacious in virtually all outcomes studied to date. TM has the greater volume of supporting research with the exception of a large volume on mindfulness, and more high-quality studies (prospective randomized controlled design) than the other two approaches (Rees, 2011; Tanner et al., 2009).

The nature of TM shifts the mind away from physical and mundane concerns to a focus on the larger universe and the individual's place within it (Maharishi Mahesh Yogi, 1999). The question I continue to ask is not who could benefit from the practice of TM, but who would not benefit from the use of TM?

References

Adler, A. B., McGurk, D., Bliese, P. D., & Hoge, C. W. (2009). Battle mind debriefing and battle mind training as early interventions with soldiers returning from Iraq: Randomization by platoon. *Journal of Consulting and Clinical Psychology, 77*(5), 928-940. doi:10.1037/a001687.

Anderson, V. L., Levinson, E. M., Barker, W., & Kiewra, K. R. (1999). The effects of meditation on teacher perceived occupational stress, state and trait anxiety, and burnout. *School Psychology Quarterly, 12*(1), 3-25.

Baldwin, C. M., Long, K. Kroesen, K., Brooks, A. J., & Bell, I. (2002). US military veterans' perception of the conventional medical care system and their use of complementary and alternative medicine. *Family Practice, 19*(1), 57-64.

Barnes, P. M., Bloom, B., & Nahin, R. L. (2008). Complementary and alternative medicine use among adults and children: United States, 2007. *National Health Statistics Report, 12*, 1-24.

Bernardi, L., Slieght, P., Bandinelli, G., Cencetti, S., Fattorini, L., Wdowcyc-Szuc, J., & Lagi, A. (2001). Effect of rosary prayer and yoga mantras on autonomic cardiovascular rhythms: Comparative study. *Behavioral Medicine Journal, 323*, 1446-1449.

Borman, J. E., Smith, T. L., Becker, S., Pada, M., Grufzinskis, A. H., & Nurmi, E. A. (2005). Efficacy of frequent mantram repetition on stress, quality of life, and spiritual wellbeing for veterans. A pilot study. *Journal of Holistic Nursing, 23*, 395-414. doi:10.1177/0898010105278929.

Borman, J. E., Golshan, S., Thorp, S. R., Wetherell, J. L., & Lang, A. J. (2009). Relationship of frequent mantram repetition to emotional and spiritual wellbeing in healthcare workers. *The Journal of Continuing Education in Nursing, 37*(5).

Borman, J. E., Golshan, S., Thorp, S. R., Wetherell, J. L., & Lang, A. J. (2009). Meditation-based mantram intervention for veterans with posttraumatic stress disorder: A randomized trial. *Psychological Trauma, Theory, Research, Practice and Policy,* 1-9. doi:10.1037/a0027522.

Borman, J. E., Liu, L., & Thorp, S. R. (2011). Spiritual wellbeing mediates PTSD change in veterans with military-related PTSD. *International Journal of Behavioral Medicine,* 497-502. doi:10.1007/s12529-011-9186-1.

Brauser, D. (2011). Just say OM: Meditation may alleviate PTSD symptoms. *Military Medicine, 176,* 626-630.

Brooks, J. S., & Scarano, T. (1985). Transcendental meditation in the treatment of post-Vietnam adjustment. *Journal of Counseling and Development, 64,* 212-215.

Cahn, R. C., Deforme, A., & Polich, J. (2010). Occipital gamma activation during Vipassana meditation. *Cognitive Process, 11,* 39-56.

Chard. K., Owens, G., & Cottingham, S. (2010). A comparison of OEF/OIF veterans and Vietnam veterans receiving cognitive processing therapy. *Journal of Traumatic Stress 23*(1), 25-32.

Chiesa, A., & Serretti, A. (2010). A systematic review of neurobiological and clinical features of mindfulness meditations. *Psychological Medicine, 40,* 1239-1252.

Chiesa, A. (2010). Vipassana meditation: Systematic review of current evidence. *The Journal of Alternative and Complementary Medicine, 16*(1), 37-46. doi:10.1089/acm.2009.0362.

Clement, C. (2005). The evocation of death anxiety on a meditation retreat. *Psychoanalysis Dialogues, 15*(2), 139-152.

REFERENCES

Cloitre, M., Courtois, C. A., Charuvastra, A., Carapezza, R., Strolbach, B. C., & Green, B. L. (2011). Treatment of complex PTSD: Results of the ISTSS expert clinician survey on best practices. *Journal of Traumatic Stress, 24*(6), 615-627.

Code of Federal Regulations (CFR) 38-62.2. Retrieved July 5, 2013, from http://www.law.cornell.edu/cfr/text/38/62.2

Collinge, W., Kahn, J., & Soltysik, R. (2012). Promoting reintegration of National Guard veterans and their partners using a self-directed program of integrative therapies: A pilot study. *Military Medicine, 177*(12), 1477-85.

Coppola, F., & Spector, D. (2009). Natural stress relief meditation as a tool for reducing anxiety and increasing self-actualization. *Social Behavior and Personality, 37*(3), 307-312. doi:10.2224/abp.2009.37.3.307.

Cukor, J., Spitalnick, J., Difede, J. A., Rizzo, A., & Rothbaum, B. O. (2009). Emerging treatments for PTSD. *Clinical Psychology Review.* doi:10.1016/j.cpr.2009.09.001.

Dillbecie, M. C. (1977). The effect of the transcendental meditation technique on anxiety level. *Journal of Clinical Psychology, 55*(4), 1076-1078.

Dillbecie, M. C., & Orme-Johnson, D. W. (1987). Psychological differences between transcendental meditation and rest. *American Psychologist, 42,* 879-881.

Elder, C., Nidich, S., Colbert, R., Hagelin, J., Grayshield, L., Oviedo-Lim, D., Nidich, R., Rainforth, M., Jones., & Gerace, D. (2008). Reduced psychological distress in racial and ethnic minority students practicing the transcendental meditation program. *Journal of Instructional Psychology, 38*(2), 109-116.

Eppley, K. R., & Abrams, A. I. (1989). Differential effects of relaxation techniques on trait anxiety: a meta-analysis. *Journal of Clinical Psychology, 45*(6), 957-974.

Everly, G. S., & Lating, J. M. (2002). A clinical guide to the treatment of human stress response, (2nd ed.). New York, NY: Kluwer Academic/Plenum Publishers.

Facts and figures on drawdown in Iraq. (2010, August 2). Retrieved October 15, 2014, from http://www.whitehouse.gov/the-press-office/facts-and-figures-drawdown-iraq

First, M. B., Frances, A., & Pincus, H. A. (2002). *DSM-IV-TR™ handbook of differential diagnosis*. Arlington, VA: American Psychiatric Publishing.

Fonata, A., Rosenheck, R., & Desi, R. (2010). Female veterans of Iraq and Afghanistan seeking care from VA's specialized PTSD programs: comparison with male veterans and female war zone veterans of previous eras. *Journal of Women's Health, 19*(4), 751-757. doi:10.1089/jwh.2009-1389.

Gaylord, C., Orme-Johnson, D., & Travis, F. (1988). The effects of the transcendental meditation technique and progressive muscle relaxation on EEG coherence, stress reactivity, and mental health in black adults. *International Journal of Neuroscience, 46,* 77-86.

Goldin, P., Wiveka, R., & Gross, J. (2009). Mindfulness meditation training and self-referential processing in social anxiety disorder: Behavioral and neural effects. *Journal of Cognitive Psychotherapy, 23*(3), 242-257. doi:10.1891/0889.23.3.242.

Grosswald, S., & Yellin, J. (2011). *The resilient warrior*. Friendswood, TX: Total Recall Publications.

Halligan, S. L., Michael, T., Wilhelm, F. H., Clark, D. M., & Ehlers, A. (2006). Reduced heart rate responding to trauma reliving in trauma survivors with PTSD: Correlates and consequences. *Journal of Traumatic Stress, 19*(5), 721-734. doi:10.1002/jts.20167.

Hamblen, Schnurr, Rosenberg, & Eftekhari. (2010). Overview of psychotherapy for PTSD. *National Center for PTSD*. Retrieved June 5, 2013, from http://www.ptsd.va.gov/professional/pages/overview-treatment-research.asp.

Hofman, S. G., Grossman, P., & Hinton, D. E. (2011). Loving-kindness and compassion meditation: Potential for psychological interventions. *Clinical Psychology Review, 31*(7), 1126-1132. doi:10.1016/j.cpr.2011.0.003.

REFERENCES

Horowitz, S. (2010). Health benefits of meditation. *Alternative and Complementary Therapies, 16*(4), 223-228. doi:10.1089/act.2012.16402.

Howard, S. (2013, April 21). Health community embraces meditation. *Honolulu Star-Advertiser,* p. A17.

Jakupcak, M., Wagner, A., Paulson, A., Varra, A., & McFall, M. (2010). Behavioral activation as a primary care based treatment for PTSD and depression among returning veterans. *Journal of Traumatic Stress, 23*(4), 491-495.

Jevning, R., Wallace, R. K., & Beidebach, M. (1992). The physiology of meditation: A review. A wakeful hypo-metabolic integrated response. *Neuroscience and Behavioral Review, 16,* 415-421.

Kearney, D. J., McDermott, K., Malte, C., Martinez, M., & Simpson, T. L. (2012). Association of participation in a mindfulness program with measures of PTSD, depression, and quality of life in a veteran sample. *Journal of Clinical Psychology 68*(1), 101-116. doi:10.1002/jclp.20853.

Klosterman, J., Rielage, Hoyt, T., & Renshaw, K. (2010). Internalizing and externalizing personality styles and psychopathology in OEF-OIF veterans. *Journal of Traumatic Stress, 23*(3), 350-357.

Kroesen, K., Baldwin, C. M., Brooks, A. J., & Bell, I. R. (2002). US military veterans' perception of the conventional medical care system and their use of complementary and alternative medicine. *Family Practice, 19*(1), 57-64.

Lang, A. J., Strauss, J. L., Bomyea, J., Borman, J. E., Hickman, S. D., Good, R. C., & Essex, M. (2012). The theoretical and empirical basis for meditation as an intervention for PTSD. *Behavior Modification, 36*(6), 759-786.

Libby, D. J., & Pilver, C. E., Desai, R. (2011). Complementary and alternative medicine use among individuals with posttraumatic stress disorder. *Psychological trauma: Theory, research, practice and policy.* doi:10.1037/a0027082.

Lord, S. (2010). Meditative dialogue: Cultivating sacred space in psychotherapy—an intersubjective fourth. *Smith College Studies in Social Work,* 80, 269-285. doi:10.1080/00377311003754187.

Macrodimitris, S. D., Hamilton, K. E., Backs-Dermott, B. J., & Mothersill, K. J. (2010). CBT basics: A group approach to teaching fundamental cognitive behavioral skills. *Journal of Cognitive Psychotherapy, 24*(2), 132-146. doi:10.1891/0889-8391.24.2.132.

Maharishi Mahesh Yogi. (1995). *Science of being and art of living/transcendental meditation.* New York, NY: Penguin Publishing.

Marchand, W. R. (2012). Mindfulness-based stress reduction, mindfulness-based cognitive therapy, and zen meditation for depression, anxiety, pain, and psychological distress. *Journal of Psychiatric Practice, 18*(4), 233-252.

Meditation programs for stress and wellbeing. Retrieved June 15, 2013, from http://www. effectivehealthcare.ahrq.gov

McAllister, T. W. (2009). Psychopharmacological issues in the treatment of TBI and PTSD. *The Clinical Neuropsychologist, 23,* 1338-1367. doi:10.1080/13854040903277289.

McLay, R. N., Loeffler, G. H., & Wynn, G. H. (2013). Research methodology for the study of complementary and alternative medicine in the treatment of military PTSD. *Psychiatric Annals, 43*(1), 38-43.

Monson, D. M., Fredman, S. J., & Adair, K. C. (2008). Cognitive-behavioral conjoint therapy for post-traumatic stress disorder: application to operation enduring and Iraqi freedom veterans. *Journal of Clinical Psychology, 64*(8), 958-971. doi:10.1002/jclp.20511.

REFERENCES

Murata, T., Takahashi, T., Hamada, T., Omori, M., Kosaka, H., Yoshida, H., & Wada, Y. (2004). Individual trait anxiety levels characterizing the properties of zen meditation. *Neuropsychobiology, 50*, 189-194. doi:10.1159/000079113.

Myers, J. E., & Young, S. J. (2012). Brain wave biofeedback: Benefits of integrating neuro-feedback in counseling. *Journal of Counseling and Development, 90*(1), 20-29.

National Institute of Health, What is complementary and alternative medicine? *National Institute of Health, National Center for Complementary and Alternative Medicine.* Retrieved June 15, 2013, from http://nccam.nih.gov

Newberg, A. B., Wintering, N., Khalsa, D. S., Roggenkamp, H., & Waldman M. R. (2012). Meditation effects on cognitive function and cerebral flood flow in subjects with memory loss: a preliminary study. *Annals of Neurosciences, 19*(2), 73-81.

Office of Public Health, VA. (2011, November 1). Public health. Retrieved August 8, 2014, from http://www.publichealth.va.gov/epidemiology

Overholser, J. C., & Fisher, L. B. (2009). Contemporary perspective on stress management: Medication, meditation or mitigation. *Journal of Contemporary Psychotherapy, 39*, 147-155. doi:10.1007/s10879-009-9114-8.

Pargament, K. I., & Sweeney, P. J. (2011). Building spiritual fitness in the army. *American Psychologist, 66*(1), 58-64. doi:10.1037/a0021657.

Pietrzak, R. H., Johnson, D. C., Goldstein, M. B., Malley, J. C., & Southwick, S. M. (2009). Perceived stigma and barriers to mental health care utilization among OEF/OIF veterans. *Psychiatric Services, 60*(8), 1118-1122.

Posadzki, P., Parekh, S., & Glass. N. (2010). Yoga and Qigong in the psychological prevention of mental health disorders: A conceptual synthesis. *Chinese Journal of Integrated Medicine, 16*(1), 80-86. doi:10.1007/s11655-009-9002-2.

Rausch, S. M., Gramling, S. E., & Auerbach, S. M. (2006). *Effects of a single session of large-group meditation and progressive muscle relaxation training on stress reduction, reactivity, and recovery*. Richmond, VA: Virginia Commonwealth University.

Rees, B. (2011). Overview of outcome data of potential meditation training for soldier resilience. *Military Medicine, 176*(11), 1232-1242.

Roberts, M., Engel, C., Cordova, E. H., & Jonas, W. (2011). Findings of VA/DoD CPG on CAM therapies for PTSD. *Defense Centers of Excellence for Psychological Health and Traumatic Brain Injury*. January 26, 2011 Military Health System Conference.

Rosenthal, N. E. (2011). *Transcendence, healing and transformation through transcendental meditation*. New York, NY: Penguin Group.

Rosenthal, J. Z., Grosswald, S., Ross, R., & Rosenthal, N. (2011). Effects of transcendental meditation in veterans of operation enduring freedom and operation Iraqi freedom with post-traumatic stress disorder: a pilot study. *Military Medicine, 176*(6), 626-630.

Saris, J., Moylan, S., Camfield, D. A., Pase, M. P., Mischoulon, D., Berk, M., Jacka, F. N., & Schweitzer, I. (2012). Complementary medicine, exercise, meditation, diet, and lifestyle modifications for anxiety disorders: A review of current evidence. *Evidence-Based Complementary and Alternative Medicine Volume, Article ID* (809653), 1-20. doi:10.1155/2012/809653.

Sayers, S. L., Farrow, V.A., Ross, J., & Oslin, D. W. (2009). Family problems among recently returned military veterans referred for a mental health evaluation. *Journal of Clinical Psychiatry, 70*(2), 163-170.

Schnurr, P. P., Kaloupek, D., Sayer, N., Weiss, D. S., Cohen, J., Galea, S., & Weaver, T. L. (2010). Understanding the impact of wars in Iraq and Afghanistan. *Journal of Traumatic Stress, 23*(1), 3-4.

Seahorn, J. S., & Seahorn, E. A. (2008). *Tears of a warrior*. Ft. Collins, CO: Team Pursuits.

REFERENCES

Seal, K. H., Bertentahl, D., Miner, C., Sauank, S., & Marmar. C. (2007). Bringing the war back home. Mental health disorders among 103,788 US veterans returning from Iraq and Afghanistan seen at department of Veterans Affairs facilities. *Archive Internal Medicine, 167,* 476-482.

Sears, S., & Kraus, S. (2009). I think therefore I Om: Cognitive distortions and coping style as meditators for the effects of mindfulness meditation on anxiety, positive and negative affect, and hope. *Journal of Clinical Psychology, 65*(6), 561-573.

Shapiro, S. L., Walsh, R., & Britton, W. B. (2003). An analysis of recent meditation research and suggestions for future directions. *Journal for Meditation and Meditation Research, 3,* 69-90.

Shea, T. M., Vujanovic, A. A., Mansfield, A. K., Sevin, E., & Liu, F. (2010). Posttraumatic stress disorder symptoms and functional impairment among OEF and OIF National Guard and reserve veterans. *Journal of Traumatic Stress, 23*(1), 100-107.

Shiner, B. (2011). Health services use in the department of veteran affairs among returning Iraq war and Afghan war veterans with PTSD. *National Center for Posttraumatic Stress Disorder Research Quarterly, 22*(2), 1-10.

Simpkins, C. A., & Simpkins, A. M. (2011). *Zen meditation in psychotherapy. techniques for clinical practice,* 135-152. Hoboken, NJ: John Wiley & Sons, Inc.

Simpson, T. L., Kaysen, D., Bowen, S., MacPherson, L. M., Chawla, N., Blume, A., Marlatt, G. A., & Larimer, M. (2007). PTSD symptoms, substance use, and vipassana meditation among incarcerated individuals. *Journal of Traumatic Stress, 20*(3), 239-249.

Strauss, J. L., & Lang, A. J. (2012). Complementary and alternative treatments for PTSD. *PTSD Research Quarterly, 23*(2), 1-7.

Tanielian, T., & Jaycox, L. H. (2008). Invisible wounds of war. Psychological and cognitive injuries, their consequences, and services to assist recovery, 87-115. *Center for Military Health Policy Research.* Santa Monica, CA: Rand Corporation.

Tanner, M. A., Travis, F., Gaylord-King, C., Haaga, D. A. F., Grosswald, S., & Schneider, R. H. (2009). The effects of transcendental meditation program on mindfulness. *Journal of Clinical Psychology, 65*(6), 574-589. doi:10.1002/jclp.20544.

Thorp, S. R., Ayers, C. R., Nuevo, R., Stoddard, J. A., Sorrell, J. T., & Wetherel, J. L. (2009). Meta-analysis comparing different behavioral treatments for late-life anxiety. *American Journal Geriatric Psychology, 17*(2), 105-115.

Toneatto, T., & Nguyen. L. (2007). Does mindfulness meditation improve anxiety and mood symptoms? A review of the controlled research. *The Canadian Journal of Psychiatry, 52*(4), 260-266.

Travis, F., & Shear, J. (2010) Focused attention, open monitoring, and automatic self-transcending: Categories to organize meditations from Vedic, Buddhist, and Chinese traditions. *Consciousness and Cognition,* doi:10.1016/jconcog 2010.01.007.

U.S. Department of Public Health. (2011) National center for health care statistics. Retrieved June 5, 2013 from http://www.cdc.gov/nchs/data

Vujanovic, A. A., Niles, B., Pietrefesa, A., Schmertz, S. K., & Potter, C. M. (2011). Mindfulness in the treatment of posttraumatic stress disorder among military veterans. *Professional Psychology, Research and Practice, 42*(1), 24-31. doi:10.1037/a0022272.

Wachholtz, A. B., & Pargament, K. I. (2005). Is spirituality a critical ingredient of meditation? Comparing the effects of spiritual meditation, secular meditation, and relaxation on spiritual, psychological, cardiac, and pain outcomes. *Journal of Behavioral Medicine, 28*(4), 369-384. doi:10.1007/s10865-005-9008-5

Wachholtz, A. B., & Pargament, K. I. (2008). Migraines and meditation: Does spirituality matter? *Journal of Behavioral Medicine, 31*, 351-356. doi:10.1007/s10865-008-9159-2.

Waelde, L. C., Uddo, M., Marquett, R., Ropelato, M., Freightman, S., Pardo, A., & Salazar, J. (2008). A pilot study of meditation for mental health workers following Hurricane Katrina. *Journal of Traumatic Stress, 21*(5), 497-500.

Wolf, D. B., & Abell, N. (2003). Examining the effects of meditation techniques on psychosocial functioning. *Research on Social Work Practice, 13*(1), 27-42.

Wood, D. P., Wiederhold, B. K., & Spira, J. (2010). Lessons learned from 350 virtual reality sessions with warriors diagnosed with combat-related posttraumatic stress disorder. *Cyberpsychology, Behavior, and Social Networking, 13*(1), 3-11. doi:10.1089/cyber.2009.0396.

Zinn, J. K., Massion, A. O., Kristeller, J., Peterson, L. G., Fletcher, K. E., Pbert, L., Lenderking, W. R., & Santorelli, S. F. (1992). Effectiveness of a meditation-based stress reduction program in the treatment of anxiety disorders. *American Journal of Psychiatry, 149*(7), 936-943.

Appendix A

Table 3

Study Types: Initial Studies Pulled vs. Final Studies Selected

Initial Finding Keywords	Initial Quantity	Final Quantity	% Comparison
Anxiety, complementary, meditation & veterans	3	1	33%
Complementary, meditation, PTSD, veterans	11	8	73%
Anxiety, complementary, meditation	6	5	83%
Complementary, meditation, PTSD	6	3	50%
Meditation, PTSD, veterans	11	4	36%
Anxiety, meditation	10	7	70%
Complementary, meditation	5	1	20%
PTSD, veterans	16	2	13%
PTSD	2	2	100%
Meditation, veteran	5	0	0%
Meditation, PTSD	4	0	0%
Complementary	1	0	0%
Meditation	8	0	0%
Veteran	0	0	0%
Total	88	33	38%

Note. Table A identifies and details the types of studies that were reviewed; it also provides additional detail on the final three studies selected and identified by keywords.

Appendix B

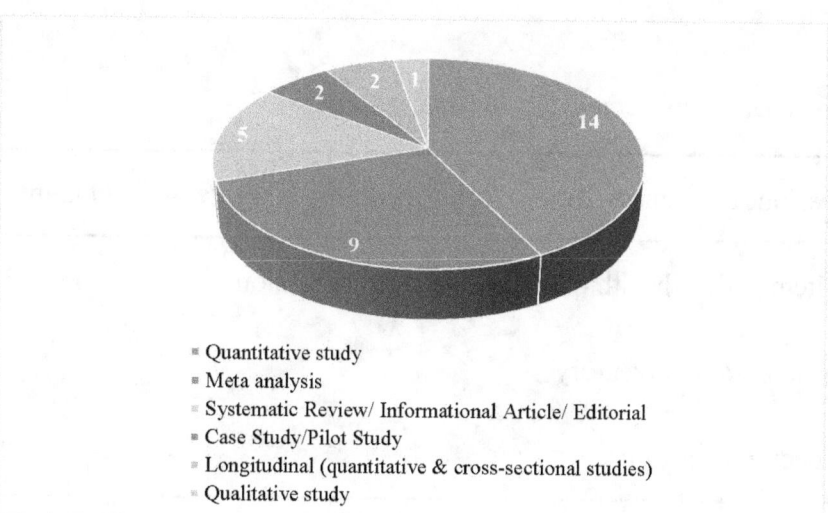

Figure 4. Study type analysis.

Note. This graph provides a comprehensive look at the various study types reviewed for this study.

Appendix C

Table 4

Health/Psychometric Measurement Tools Used in Studies

No.	Depression Assessment Tool	Quantity Of Use
1	Nine-item patient health questionnaire for depression	1
2	Becks depression inventory	7
	Total occurrences of use	8

Note: 46 Psychometric tools used 77 total times in 33 studies.

Table 5

PTSD Assessment Tools Quantity of Use

No.	PTSD Assessment Tool	Quantity Of Use
1	Clinically administered PTSD scale	3
2	Combat exposure scale	1
3	PTSD checklist civilian	2
4	PTSD checklist-military version	4
	Total occurrences of use	10

Table 6

Health/Physical Assessment Tools Quantity of Use

No.	Health/Physical Assessment Tool	Quantity of Use
1	Demographic and health-related variables	1
2	Electrochocardiogram(EKG)	4
3	Electroencephalogram (EEG).brain wave	1
4	Health survey short form (SF-12)	1
5	Heart rate variability	1
6	Medical symptom checklist	1
7	Objective measurements of pain tolerance	1
8	Screened for alcohol abuse	1
9	Screened for domestic abuse	1
10	Self-report surveys	2
11	Talairach and Tournoux coordinates of maximum BOLD signal intensity voxel	1
12	Surveys	1
	Total occurrences of use	16

Table 7

Anxiety Assessment Tools Quantity of Use

No.	Anxiety Assessment Tool	Quantity of Use
1	Beck anxiety inventory	1
2	Liebowitz social anxiety inventory	1
3	Perceived stress scale	2
4	Rumination style questionnaire	1
5	Speilberger state trait inventory-anxiety and anger	4
6	The state-trait anxiety inventory for adults	5
7	The teacher stress inventory	1
8	Trait disassociation questionnaire	1
	Total occurrences of use	16

Table 8

Psychiatric Assessment Tools Quantity of Use

No.	Psychiatric Assessment Tools	Quantity of Use
1	16 personality factor questionnaire	1
2	Clinicians global impression severity scale	1
3	Clinicians global impression-improvement scales	2
4	Critical incident interview method (qualitative)	1
5	Daily diary	1
6	Functional assessment on chronic ill therapy spiritual wellbeing scale	2
7	Maslach burnout inventory	1
8	Mini-international psychiatric interview	1
9	Positive/negative affect scale	1
10	Quality of life enjoyment and satisfaction questionnaire	4
11	RAND Corporation 1-9 rating scale to assess the appropriateness of a technique	1
12	Rosenberg self-esteem scale	1
13	Spiritual wellbeing scale	3
14	Brief system inventory-18	1
15	NCS-R	1
16	NLAAS	1
17	NSAL surveys. See article for acronym definitions	1
18	The symptom checklist-90-revised	1
19	CPES	1
20	Self-rating scales and ratings of trained interviewers	1
	Total occurrences of use	27

Note. The tables in Appendix C provide a comprehensive review of the various American Psychiatric Association-approved psychometric measuring instruments used in the studies reviewed.

Appendix D

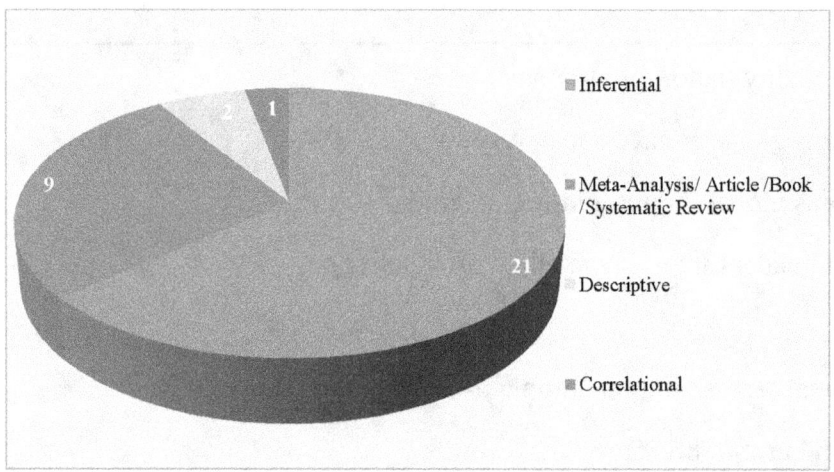

Figure 5. Statistical data summary.

Note. This graph provides a comprehensive overview of the statistical data analyses the researchers used in their studies.

Epilogue

Tightness in my stomach. Talk about anxiety. I had just spent the previous month and a half preparing my oral defense of the study that was the foundation of this book. 30 minutes into the defense, and I could see the light at the end of the tunnel. The culminating event of over five years of reading, research, writing and re-writing was about to be completed when, in a casual suggestion, someone wondered what the "current research" (within the last year two years), held in the way of support for my study. I immediately played over in my head the thought of having to rewrite, yet again, my study to include research that had been conducted since completing the gathering of the research used as the foundation of my study. Tightness in my stomach which represented the anxiety associated with the realization that the light at the end of the tunnel was not daylight but an on-coming train. At least that is what it felt like that morning. Once I got over my mad, and begun the task of rolling up my sleeves and getting down to answering the boards inquiry regarding recent research that supports my study, I actually began to feel encouraged.

What I found were numerous comprehensive studies that were conducted in 2013 and 2014 that more than supported the concept that meditation has measurable positive effects on reducing the psychological and physiological side effects of stress and trauma.

Fortunately, after a thorough evaluation of what else was required I deduced that my study did not have to be re-written. I wanted to share with the reader current evidence based and exciting empirical studies that were from 2013 and 2014 that speak to the positive effects of meditation for people seeking help with managing the negative effects of anxiety.

Of note, was a study done and published in the (*Journal of Traumatic Stress,* Aug, 2014, 27, pp. 397-406) titled "Breathing-Based Meditation decreases Posttraumatic Stress Disorder

Symptoms in US Military Veterans: A randomized controlled longitudinal study, by Ema Seppala et al. In this study, the authors concluded that given that the debilitating impact of PTSD on our returning Veterans, and the limited success of current interventions (ie: CPT, PE, EMDR and pharmacological) there is a critical need to expand, for the Veterans, the range of treatment intervention options available. The breathing based meditation in this study showed positive improvements on psychophysiological and symptom measures. In other words, it had positive impact on the reduction of negative symptoms of PTSD in military veterans such as, elevated heart rates and the reduction of hyper arousal symptoms.

Similarly, the study titled Significant Reductions in Posttraumatic Stress Symptoms in Congolese Refugees Within 10 Days of Transcendental Meditation Practice, (*Journal of Traumatic Stress*, 27, 2014, pp,112-115). As suggested by the title, this study looked at the effects of practicing TM twice a day with refugees who lived in the Congo and experienced various forms of trauma associated with war and victimization. The study found that within 30 days of learning and practicing the Transcendental Meditation Program, study participants became non-symptomatic of high levels of PTSD symptoms. A significant finding in this study was that the non-TM technique control group remained at the same high level of PTSD symptoms throughout the entire 135 day test.

Lastly, a meta-analysis conducted by David W. Orme-Johnson, PhD, and Vernon A. Barnes, PhD, titled Effects of the Transcendental Meditation Technique on Trait Anxiety: a meta-analysis of randomized controlled trials (*The Journal of Alternative and Complementary Medicine,* 19(0), 2013, pp. 1-12) was a very significant meta-analysis. In this meta-analysis over 600 TM research papers were identified, and 14 of these address trait-anxiety that included 1295 participants with diverse demographic characteristics. The findings showed that the TM practice is more effective than treatment as usual and most other treatments, with the greatest effects observed in individuals with high anxiety.

EPILOGUE

In keeping with the proposal of my study regular transcendental meditation practice in populations of patients with chronic anxiety, veterans with PTSD, and prison inmates along with people diagnosed with high blood pressure, and at risk for heart attack and stroke as a result of stress and anxiety showed significant reductions in the negative psychological and physiological effects of anxiety within the mind and body.

About the Author

Dr. Martin has an exemplary clinical career working with the military and their families. For over twenty-five-years he has done private practice, directed and managed multiple outpatient programs in federal, state, and private health care settings.

He has over 25 years of experience as a clinical psychotherapist, and currently practices out of his office in Aiea, HI, and lives with his Ohana in Mililani, HI. As a cognitive behavioral therapist he specializes in treating soldiers, and their families dealing with stress related issues resulting from deployment(s) and reintegration issues. He also specializes in conflict management with adults, marital issues, chemical dependency, anxiety, depression and trauma issues.

Dr. Martin was recognized as the NASW Hawaii Clinician of the Year in 2012, He specializes in Cognitive Behavioral Therapy, and trauma therapy as a treatment modality to help clients that are current, or previous Military Service Members. He believes that there are behaviors that can't be controlled through rational thought, but emerge based on prior conditioning from the environment, and other external, and/or internal stimuli. He helps clients to be "problem focused" and "action oriented".

He helps them select specific strategies that can address their problems, and help them determine courses of action, and achieve personal and professional goals by unlocking their full potential. When our brains are healthy, he believes that "it is our thinking that causes us to feel and act the way we do".

Dr.Martin helps individuals, families, and couples in therapy view obstacles in their lives as opportunities, and believes they, ultimately, make the decision to change, or not in their lives. He helps them to recognize destructive patterns of thinking and reacting, and help them to modify, or replace them.

He feels that if we experience unwanted feelings and behaviors, then we need to identify the thinking that is causing them, and learn how to replace this thinking with thoughts that lead to outcomes that are more desirable.

Thanks to modern technology, I work with clients from around the world helping them navigate their journey of healing, and helping them effect change in their lives.

Change is hard for any of us. However, people often value consistency over happiness because they fear change more than they desire to be happy. If we cannot see ourselves outside of our own aquariums we cannot get a perspective and develop insight into what behavior(s) that need to change to be healthy and happy.

I have found meditation to be instrumental to this end. Introspection is one of the greatest gifts we can give ourselves and those in our lives that we care about and are connected to.

The Journey inward continues............